UNLOCKING
Frozen Shoulder

UNLOCKING
Frozen Shoulder

A New Paradigm of Treatment

L Y N N   V A R C I N

BALBOA
PRESS

A DIVISION OF HAY HOUSE

Art Credit: Peter Letts & John Daryl D. Obera, RN

Balboa Press books may be ordered through booksellers or by contacting:

Balboa Press
A Division of Hay House
1663 Liberty Drive
Bloomington, IN 47403
www.balboapress.com.au
1-(877) 407-4847

ISBN: 978-1-4525-1072-9 (sc)
ISBN: 978-1-4525-1073-6 (e)

The information, ideas, and suggestions in this book are not intended as a substitute for professional medical advice. Before following any suggestions contained in this book, you should consult your personal physician. Neither the author nor the publisher shall be liable or responsible for any loss or damage allegedly arising as a consequence of your use or application of any information or suggestions in this book.

A fear of being sued is associated with the trend in our society to overzealously look to place blame on others. This book is the antithesis of that; it is about looking inside yourself to help your own pain and stiffness. It is more than just a matter of being positive, as it involves beginning movements yourself at home. There are precautions specific to exercise, particularly for readers with joint problems or joint replacements. Read diligently and exercise softly; it is all about self-healing and not harm.

Balboa Press rev. date: 09/25/2013

Dedicated to all those who care more.

When you open a receptor, ensure *love* is the energy that sustains.

CONTENTS

A LITTLE ABOUT THE AUTHOR

In addition to holding qualifications in physiotherapy and ergonomics from the Universities of Sydney and Queensland (Australia), Lynn Varcin has completed post-graduate master studies in philosophy and metaphysics. She is also a trained Therapeutic Touch™ and Feldenkrais™ Practitioner. She has extensive professional experience in both the public and private sectors. When Lynn herself began to suffer from frozen shoulder, she initially took a traditional scientific approach to treatment, addressing only the physical aspects of the condition. However, as the disorder progressed from one shoulder to the next, Lynn became aware that emotional factors contributed to the condition. Based on this recognition she began to wonder if empathy and willingness to hear stories from her own client's *[talking about their emotional and social trauma(s)]* naturally aided their recovery more than she had previously comprehended. Out of these personal and professional experiences and observations Lynn developed the holistic theory and approach presented in *Unlocking Frozen Shoulder: A new paradigm in treatment*. This became a journey through hormonal disbalance with adhesive capsulitis, and inadvertently finding a probable cause of primary frozen shoulder. Lynn lives in Byron Bay, Australia. Her work in Indigenous Healthcare continues as a physiotherapist but her passion remains in promoting life coaching actions for internal healing practices in difficult to diagnose and treat conditions. Exercises in the book vary from traditional approaches and as such set her aside from most therapists prescribing stretching and pendular shoulder exercises.

THE STORY OF A LAKE
A PARABLE

There once was a strong stream that fed a beautiful lake. The lake's owner loved to stand on its shore and enjoy its beauty. Five tributaries supported the stream. One day, mud was stirred up in one of the tributaries. The other tributaries worked hard to cleanse the stream before it could contaminate the waters of the lake, because those waters were precious, irreplaceable—except, of course, by God.

Yet the muddied tributary continued to work itself into a mess; unable to calm the turbulent mud, in its distress it pumped up even more. The stream itself resisted the mud and changed directions, affecting the surrounding shore. The owner stood on the shore and gazed across the lake, unaware of the numerous small chain reactions occurring beneath the surface.

Now the mud began backing up into another tributary. There was no back-flow valve, and the mud was soon spreading the length of the second tributary.

The lake settled into its new situation, adapting quickly, breeding chains of chemicals to prevent pollution, but the original tributary continued to feed mud into the stream, which began to dry out. Its flow was no longer alterable. The second tributary, damaged upstream, began to slow more and more. Hard physical activity was needed to clean that stream, but the owner, stunned by the sudden and unexpected changes in the lake, could only stand by helplessly. A third tributary started to act in a preventive capacity, but the water rate had now slowed to a trickle.

The lake adapted again, reacting well to the new input. The owner stood on the shore, dreaming of all five tributaries functioning well again soon. But now one tributary had frozen, and farther upstream harm continued, unnoticed by the owner who could only feel the freeze.

CHAPTER 1

THE FROZEN SHOULDER

Also, all knowledge seems to be teachable,
and what is known is learnable.
Aristotle

Frozen shoulder is also called *adhesive capsulitis, capsulitis,* and *primary or secondary frozen shoulder.* It normally takes two years to heal. The term *itis* means inflammation; *capsule* is the name of the tissue involved—hence *capsul-itis.* It can affect anyone and has no known cause. The arm becomes extremely painful, and then, often suddenly the movements at the shoulder also begin to tighten, or "adhere." This affects your ability to move, turn your forearm, and lift your arm. Frozen shoulder is very debilitating; many physical therapists believe it is one of the most difficult conditions to fix. Few can stop the freezing stage once it has commenced. Worse still is that you may additionally begin to have capsulitis on the opposite shoulder after six to twelve months of the other one repairing itself. So keep reading!

The American Shoulder and Elbow Surgeons define frozen shoulder as *"a condition of uncertain etiology characterized by significant restriction of both active and passive shoulder motion that occurs in the absence of a known intrinsic shoulder disorder."* (Hsu et al., 2010, pp 502)

The arm can ache, or twinge prior to really acute pain. There may be a hot spot in one area of the arm or a tender patches over the joint area. There is usually no recollection of one specific injury that could result in this amount of pain. Tissue takes six weeks to heal, but this injury goes on for months and months, even with appropriate therapeutic interventions. When ignored it progresses to extreme loss of range of movement: the arm cannot be lifted sideways at all. Some women say it is more painful than having a baby, and we should know! Even the neck, shoulder, and back muscles begin to ache in their efforts to compensate for the lack of range. Sleeping is problematic and mood swings common.

Frozen shoulder is not linked specifically to any occupation or genetic disposition. Statistics reported in medical journals indicate that frozen shoulder affects up to 5 percent of the population (higher in diabetic populations) and is more common in women over forty years of age. Frozen shoulder continues to baffle medical practitioners, who consistently report that frozen shoulder is of unknown etiology. This means there is no known specific cause. Controversy surrounds the effectiveness of various physical and medical treatments relating to this shoulder condition. Time remains the single most efficient healer of the condition, and—sorry to say—it takes two to three years! Whether or not other body systems remain in *disbalance** is a matter for longer-term study. *[*Disbalance is intentionally used throughout the book, as unbalanced implies unhinged or mentally affected in Australian slang.]*

An intricate system is involved in frozen shoulder, and within this book I propose a new model for more successful healing and outcomes. The condition is thought to start most commonly as a vague, intermittent pulling sensation or discomfort, usually around the shoulder tendon areas. A gripping sensation precursors the stiffening phase. It is often ignored or wrongly attributed to an injury of the rotator cuff, the system of muscles and tendons that stabilize the shoulder. The actual cause, however, is an underlying stress causing messenger and receptor imbalances in the body. The balance inside your system has become undone.

To date, this has only been alluded to in some journal articles noting the abnormally high incidence of frozen shoulder in people with diabetes and thyroid dysfunctions (high and low). Within the book reference is made to hormones, connective tissue, and the nervous system and unique exercises and tasks as fascinating as they are tough to perform. If you are game to read on and self-discover the cause, then your arm pain and frozen shoulder are not going to have the standard two-year recovery rate. Healing will be accomplished much faster, depending more on your own needs and the initiation of a self-care program.

A joint threatened will be braced. Pain will stop use of the arm while the body braces the shoulder back into itself. The capsular adhesions represent a tightening in different areas, which unfortunately result in a loss of range of movement or *freeze*. All movements become extremely difficult and are very painful.

The outline of care in this book is a result of my own experiences and the fact that traditional therapies failed to heal my pain or range of movement. As a practicing physical therapist and Feldenkrais practitioner I disliked being on the receiving end of ineffective costly therapy treatments. The program began after studying Metaphysics and re-learning meditation and affirmation variances. It was quite crazy to get in touch with inner knowledge or higher consciousness initially. The first time you actually hear something you cannot possibly know, it is shocking; especially for someone trained in more traditional western medicine models. To be truthful I actually panicked, jarred my shoulder, and booked scans. And I certainly stopped meditating for a while, too. After some scans to eliminate the presence of a tumor, I discovered I was being supplied with incredible information for frozen shoulder solutions, for a variety of conditions. So the approach contained here includes not only getting you to relate hormones, mood, and your emotional history to the shoulder, but also has some really different, weird-looking movements. (I use the term *movements* instead of *exercises* as I am not into pain or drama.)

These movements are totally different to my previous knowledge; it can be hard to comprehend how getting into a froglike position has anything to do with frozen shoulder at all, but wait until you see the results. While I initially assumed some exercises to be some type of fascial stretching or nerve stretch, I continued to observe that older bodies could get into this position without the harm I would have imagined. The expansion of this experience is the source of the knowledge presented in this book. It remains new and unused in clinical trials, like many techniques.

The release of hormones and related chemical messengers on the limbic-hypothalamic-pituitary-adrenal axis (LHPA) deserves more study in relation to this shoulder condition. This complex system is a major player in linking emotions, mood, and energy reserves at a cellular level. The affect from emotional causes is even more dramatic amongst those already challenged in this axis. This includes those with pituitary problems, diabetes, and hormone insufficiencies (e.g., adrenocorticotropic hormone, or ACTH) and probably perimenopausal states. Whether or not the menopause can be considered a pre-existing deficiency is debatable. Perhaps the menopausal changes in needs, mood, and emotional reactions makes this group more vulnerable to tissue changes by altered levels of cortisol, a catabolic hormone that can weaken tissue over a long term. (*Catabolic* means simply breaking down complex molecules into simpler ones in order to release energy.) For me, especially in hindsight, it was a specific emotional stressor that was catastrophic. Dealing with these deficiencies requires separate interventions and transgresses from traditional approaches to the condition of frozen shoulder.

Mental processes affect mood, and certain stressors can be reversed with cognition and physical hard work. Whether or not the time associated with the healing of a frozen shoulder can be foreshortened depends on the release of hormones involved. **As behaviors and reactions affect all hormones, fear has to be considered the prime cause of this condition.** People (and some animals) freeze when frightened. How can this relate to you, then? For example, the stress-related hormone ACTH discharged in extreme emotional circumstances can lead to tissue laxity through the overproduction of catabolic steroids. How that laxity affects someone is dependent also on preexisting muscular length and on the joint surface condition. For example, in diabetes there are already collagen changes that exist locally. This will naturally affect tissue tolerance and shoulder strength at the capsular level. Another person may, however, experience a different physiological response, such as indigestion, emotional overeating, or high blood pressure.

In devising treatment one should consider the individual's social, emotional, and genetic disposition as part of a thorough medical history. Can one consultant do this? In fact, it is outside the scope of any one practitioner to heal a shoulder injury of this type. Many people rely on exercise and mobilization with a physical therapist. It is important to consider the reason for the freeze in the first place.

Surgical interventions are no different. Surgery can alter the person's short-term shoulder outcomes. But is it better medical practice to heal the signs or the cause? Could frozen shoulder be one of many precursors to an ongoing limbic-hypothalamic-pituitary-adrenal axis (LHPA) system in *disbalance*? Perhaps the physical body can return to a new functioning homeostasis (balance); with or without surgical or therapeutic interventions. Noting, any stress of a similar nature may heighten a similar component in the LHPA system and lead to more or other stress-related disorders *(e.g., digestive disorders, chest pain, blood pressure)*.

Assume an open-minded approach to this condition. Testing imbalances in hormones is difficult, with results variable even over a twenty-four hour period. Support your medical practitioners with the following:

- Write up a full and thorough history of any emotionally charged events as well as presence or absence of any physical harm, injury, repetitious movements, sports, or jobs you hate
- When no physical indicator is present explore logically any emotionally charged reasons or events that keep you in a nonresolved state.
- Check if any of the following prewarning signs were present (try to recall to the best of your ability).
  ➤ sensations of being overwhelmed (six months prior)

> strong sensations or feelings of rejection or hopelessness related to recollection of retrenchment, financial loss, or separation *[it is the authors opinion that feelings of rejection left unchecked alter hormonal pathways in a narrow band somehow influencing this particular shoulder condition]*

> feeling morose or hopeless or unusually sad, etc. (six to nine months prior)

> dull ache prior to pain and before night pain

> squeezing of upper arm automatically (around the deltoid) in attempt to give pain relief (limbic system response before the freeze)

> intermittent local tendon pain or pulling or tugging or other random sensations in the shoulder area well before the acute pain phase (*disbalance* sign)

> stress (emotional *disbalance*)

> reacting to any event in a hyperactive or hypersensitive way (emotional *disbalance*)

> sensations of fatigue unrelated to physical events (physical *disbalance*)

> hate, laughter, and overwhelming sensations of sadness atypical to your personality (emotional *disbalance*)

Using these criteria as a diagnostic guide is helpful but insufficient; further study on the mix of emotional and physical signs needs to be undertaken with an expert. Each person has a chance to reverse his or her own emotional traumas through altering reactions or perceptions. Where the trauma is addressed professionally with physical therapy alone, ensure a program of self-help is implemented to cover any residue LHPA system involvement.

While the limbic-hypothalamic-pituitary-adrenal axis (LHPA) access is proposed as the key, there are other brain areas and neuro anatomical links that disbalance for emotional reasons. These are the upstream complications referred to in the parable. For example fear or anxiety are said to upset balance in the central amygdala altering neuropeptides, glutamate and many other neuromodulators (Panksepp, 2001, pp147) [*]. This book deals with shoulders that are reversible in their injury status. Most are able to reverse receptor sensitivity with training and time. The use of biofield therapies can add a new treatment dimension for emotional factors relating to neural receptor chains, research is emerging in this area too slowly due to skepticism.

Can you imagine there is an emotional layer around and within you communicating with your physical body and able to alter all hormones and potentiate new neural balance. I need you to understand that as truth to believe in your own body, as often after the emotional turmoil you are going through the body develops a system of coping without hearing. The emotional needs are a system available to the hormone whisperer. The emotions are not necessarily comprehended in logic. They need not be. The emotion you are accessing here is only the one affecting the arm pain. If the arm pain were not part of the emotional system then it will be better in 5-8 working weeks, ok? I am going to call this layer of energy emotional SEL.

Panksepp J., 2001. *The Neuro-evolutionary Cusp between emotions and cognitions. Evolution and Cognition, 7 (2): 141-163.*

CHAPTER 2

INTRODUCING THE TERM *SEL*

Spontaneous healings, psychic phenomena, amazing feats of strength and endurance, the ability to walk across hot coals without getting burned, acupuncture's ability to diminish pain by moving chi around the body, and many other paranormal phenomena defy Newtonian biology.
Bruce Lipton

The book contains a new word: *SEL*. *SEL* is not to be confused with *cell*. The human body, for example, has 100 trillion cells varying in size and complexity. *SEL is a cluster of energy substances around and in the human being.* It is capitalized to emphasize that it is a newly coined term and to eliminate spelling confusions. SEL is contained by energy fields around you. SEL should not be confused with auras or auric fields; it is the content layers and frequency thereof.

SEL is a group of atoms of information, or banding waves, that form in around the body. SEL responds to stimuli and reacts very similarly to a single cell but does not contain the organelles found within cells. SEL attracts energy, disperses, and can be stagnant in time and space (this is complex but apparently very helpful in understanding intergenerational traumas in the future). SEL is not visible nor to date scientifically acknowledged; it is considered by some to be the aura and the linking energy, or etheric layer. One may expand it into band waves or frequencies or even more formal groupings related to its action, such as spiritual SEL, physical SEL, emotional SEL, and the eternal soul SEL.

For the course of this book, SEL groupings are assumed to have receptors and feedback mechanisms and operate in a transitionary plane. There is, for example, a body of *emotional SEL* that incorporates all your feelings and locked memories. Emotional SEL can be seen only if acted out through the *physical SEL* affecting the physical body, e.g., stress, crying, or even running away or freezing in fear. *Spiritual* and *soul SEL* is all about God or the *I am,* and as important as that is, it will not be covered in this book. It affects pain too; ask someone who has been mistreated in the name of God. This book will focus on an innovative way of resolving a hard-to-diagnose-and-treat shoulder condition that remains at the boundary of understanding.

The foundation of this new book on shoulder pain is that it offers three possible gateways to relate healing and injury mechanisms, each relating to SEL:

1. Natural weakening of shoulder tissue and a new "abnormal" position of the ball-and-socket joint, leading to micro-trauma. This is naturally physical SEL related and will require exercise, joint compression and self-evaluation of posture and motion.
2. Being rejected or continually not believed/acknowledged/ honored by those you love, resulting in a negative attitude to one's own self over a long period of time, depression, and altered hormones. You exceed your own SEL tolerance.
3. Problems in, within, or preexisting in the limbic-hypothalamic-pituitary-adrenal axis.

The theory implied is that any trauma or distress of significance will impact the chemical messengers linking the emotional and physical SELs. This includes the belief that emotional SEL is able to alter the peptides and chemical messengers, thus potentially altering physical SEL from standard operations. I am proposing emotion as outside energy.

I have to take the liberty to assume you believe that your body extends outside its layer of skin in the form of frequency emissions. An odd way of confirming this is to allow someone you dislike to stand too close to you; even though they are not touching, what do you sense? Is it only an encroachment into *your space?* Some people even get goose-bump warning of bad SEL. Another way is to be near someone you really love and sense a *connection*.

Each layer uses conglomerates of energy. It may be emotions, reactions, and perception, nonetheless the term *emotional SEL* is used for the purpose of *hormone whispering*. You can alter emotional SEL reactions and perception and as a consequence heal your pain and shoulder range of movement faster. **This is another key to unlocking frozen shoulder.**

Currently your physical SEL is hurting, but to what extent is the invisible emotional SEL clogged with harmful emotions, reactions, and perceptions that continue to affect your being? The use of certain mental processes to unclog this is possible with practice. Your body can naturally and gently learn to listen to its intuitive SELf for what it needs.

Emotional SEL can be altered from inside out (*e.g., hormone whispering*) with an energy-based treatment approach such as Therapeutic Touch™ and quite possibly by natural healers who work with energy fields. The power of the mind can alter neurochemical messaging; each of the aforementioned modalities alters tissue in the shoulder in a way that is separate and totally differently to what is conceived in current physical therapy mechanisms.

CHAPTER 3

YOUR SHOULDER

It is sense-perception alone that is adequate for grasping the particulars.
Aristotle

Pain is affected by your emotional SEL. Pain is a message from your body telling you to *listen*. Sometimes pain is there due to nerve-ending stress. Pain is affected by genetic factors, emotional overlay, and your own body's ability to block messages. When you are not listening the right way, pain will make tissues alter, movements change, joint positions vary. This is the situation you find yourself in with frozen shoulder or any capsular syndrome. I propose this theory.

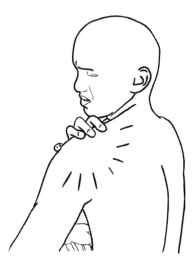

Shoulder Joint Position

The release of catabolic hormones (e.g., from stress) weakens muscular tissues supporting the shoulder. The *ball* within the shoulder joint changes position, which leads to injury in tissues from simple movements. When the capsule slackens or joint laxity occurs, and with subtle separation, the pain can begin a discomfort and intermittent ache. Depending on which muscles have weakened more, other muscles groups may contribute to rotational abnormalities, too. Inappropriate use of an *aging* arm, weakened through the action of the catabolic hormones, will eventually exhibit night pain if a balance cannot be created in the physical body. The natural belief is that it will just go away on its own.

Once this *disbalance* becomes more serious, the body will automatically respond in a variety of ways, including tightening of the capsular gap through an inflammatory response/adhesion formation, and varying other polypeptide production to account for increasing amounts of cortisol and other messenger chemicals. Sometimes, this becomes extremely painful. This pain and any other symptoms, such as swelling and patches of heat, are your body's way of warning you that worse is yet to come. If the pain is ignored, the range of movement decreases rapidly. A local vascularization between the capsular layers is, contrary to medical belief, an absolutely ingenious bodily response, as the shoulder joint literally adheres itself back into the socket. To maintain its new strength, like any freshly applied gluey mass, it wants to stay in place to ensure tightness for the future. The classic prognosis for frozen shoulder is a two—to three-year spontaneous recovery. This period is perhaps the time the body needs to regenerate enough balance between movement and fixation, and purposely "maladapt." Frozen shoulder is literally a brilliant *mal*adjustment, and an effort to keep the ball up in the socket.

Understanding What Happened to Your Arm

It is more than likely that you had symptoms before the shoulder pain started. One of the common identifiers to a hormonally based cause of frozen shoulder is having had significant emotional stress up to six months before the *freeze*. Another is diabetes.

The event has to have major impact on your nervous system, be easy to remember, or maintain a lingering charged emotional memory. For the purpose of unlocking your freeze the event will be referred to as the *emotional trauma*. The *emotional trauma* can be from any source or trauma (e.g., job loss, death of a loved one, separation). Often, this bad emotional trauma may easily stimulate negative behavioral patterns in your day-to-day life, such as sadness, depression, negative self-talk, or guilt. **There is a cascade of hormones, chemical messengers, and responsive reactions over a period of time that causes changes in and around the body prior to the onset of tissue damage.** That this eventually leads to frozen shoulder additionally indicates a certain physical lack in the upper body. Physical lack implies joint *disbalance*. *Disbalance* in this application is where one side is allowed to change the direction of movement. Combined with joint asymmetry, be it from long-time neglect or hormonally driven middle-age changes, the joint is vulnerable. **Chemistry and exercise are the two keys required in abundance to prevent and unlock your frozen shoulder.**

Secondary frozen shoulders are traditionally considered to have originated from a tear or misuse phenomenon in the tendons of the shoulder. I disagree. There is unlikely to have been trauma without some degree of *disbalance* in the glenohumeral (shoulder) joint first. Frozen shoulders that respond to treatment are such cases. Frozen shoulders that are nonresponsive to treatment fit the pattern of time healing better than any other intervention over a two-year period.

But any significant emotional trauma while any shoulder tissue is repairing makes full-blown frozen shoulder a more likely event. Therefore, a little fight back will be necessary to initiate hormonal changes posttrauma. The strategy presented here for unlocking frozen shoulder uses *hormone whispering*. *Hormone whispering* is a mindful approach to what your body needs in that instant. For example, does it need ice or warmth? How many repetitions of that exercise are needed? And so on. Your unconscious needs are taught to surface into understanding, thoughts, or sudden insight. The body itself adapts quickly to the strategy; your body will always want to move itself towards physical and emotional homeostasis or love. If there is significant lack of love, your emotional SEL will shift further, thereby altering an unknown homeostasis.

Your own body is naturally driven to heal itself, independent of any medical or therapeutic interventions. *Hormone whispering* is simply going to access a super highway into your consciousness to speed up an otherwise long healing time. Your unconscious self will remember things you are blocking. Using any system that unblocks these safely is a key to unlocking the process, too.

Hormones

Hormones are one type of chemical messenger. Hormones are released by tissues at various places in the body and affect target areas. Hormones circulate throughout the body; some can affect the brain, while others act locally on tissues.

The adrenal cortex releases glucocorticoids following times of prolonged stress. A history of emotional trauma can engender sensations of rejection, hopelessness, and inability to change the situation. The reaction mechanism here is different from the faster *flight-or-fight* hormonal releases. The hypothalamus is involved. The hypothalamus is the part of the brain that links the nervous system to the endocrine system. This system is extremely powerful and can activate and affect most organs in the body directly or indirectly.

Physical Trauma and Emotional Trauma

Physical trauma: If you had a mechanical injury, perhaps there is a micro-tear in capsular tissue, tendons, or at the joint. Diagnosis is common at the rotator cuff or the biceps tendon. The capsule in the shoulder joint literally holds the two shoulder bones, the ball and socket, together. The shoulder capsule is made up of many layers. If the multiple layers of muscles (rotator-cuff muscles and biceps, triceps, etc.) are weakened, then the weight of the arm tends to hang off other tissues a little more than it should. Consequently, when you reach or turn your arm back (or out), it can catch painfully. This, by the way, is an early hint that a little more strength to hold the joint into its socket is required urgently. (The Shoulder CPR exercises in Chapter 7 help with this.)

Why, then, is your shoulder getting worse, and freezing up? Be aware that a state of shoulder dysfunction makes a physical strain more likely to occur. This can stem from physical disability or something as bizarre as long-term self-loathing and consequent lack of exercise. Menopause and diabetes play a role in tissue asymmetry, too. For both of these conditions, it is relevant to examine the *hormone whispering* in light of local tissue strength. Use the exercises from chapter 7 carefully but as soon as possible. Diet is extremely important for both menopausal women and diabetics: improve your diet appropriately with more fish and a little more sun (for cutaneous synthesis of Vitamin D). Ensure your medical practitioner or endocrinologist understands all your moods, actions, and reactions and prescribes a hormone replacement or balancer for only as long as necessary, as links to altered perception with *hormone whispering* can be enough to alter uptake of what is naturally there.

Emotional trauma: If you had a significant emotional event a minimum of three months before arm discomfort, this will already have altered the tissues. To what degree tissues will be affected on a longer term will vary depending on your mental state and associated reactions, perception, memory, etc. If, for example, the event was tragic, but inconsequential to everything else, your recovery will be enabled only by your ability to put this tragedy in a perspective that is safe. Perhaps distractions and denial work for some, but for most it is time and more time. Do you feel any link to the frozen shoulder yet?

If on the other hand the emotional trauma was separation from some person you loved significantly and everything about that relationship interfered with all aspects of your life, then that's going to take time. Emotions that are raw over a widespread path will affect hormones dangerously, even affecting liver fatty deposits, blood pressure, tissue weakness, insulin receptors, etc. The shoulder muscles weaken, too. If you experienced a significant long-lasting emotional trauma, the pain can be as acute as a blow. An emotional trauma creates a condition of imbalance, in response to which polypeptides, hormones, and other chemicals pour out to assist. The body is brilliant in its perfection at any point in time. As you provide different emotional and chemical inputs (e.g., dietary), the body will use whatever it has inside to bring about a different set of chemical messengers to restore balance.

Sometimes, the normal messengers are not available in sufficient numbers to battle long-term, low- to middle-grade stress. That is when hormones like cortisol take over the function of organs such as the liver. These chemical messengers can take months to restore. The body in the mean time will seek a new balance another way and wipe out another peptide group, as time and time again it is trying to get you to "hear" (i.e., "Stop, rest, and fix me, please."). The *hormone whispering* targets the body's need to listen and with practice assumes you will change chemical pathways. Lacking in the right compounds, the ability of the body to manufacture new, perfect solutions decreases with time. On this basis, I provide dietary advice to my clients following simple raw food guidelines like this: feed your system with fresh organic produce as often as possible, avoiding herbicides and plastic products that are heated. Even more importantly, take away your stressor, and definitely avoid people who are negative about anything! The adrenal activity is complex, so people reading this who have diabetes may be able to influence emotional trauma but have to be even more vigilant with sugar and processed foods.

What Is the Link Between the Emotional Trauma and the Pain?

The body has a lot of checks and balances. Often the system is affected by thoughts or recollections, and this alters chemical discharges and hormones.

Interestingly the body was born with only a certain amount of ability to make any hormone a certain way. When the body lacks that particular hormone, it will add balance through stimulation of other neurochemicals and chemical messenger releases. Imagine a well-designed system being neglected or run down in ONE area, and then other areas needing to compensate.

The trouble is these hormones are related to other bodily actions. So as the behavior or trauma is allowed to continue, more organs become involved. In this case your shoulder tissue is not the only organ. Hormones have internal and external feedback loops and links; they alter shape and sensitivity and react cleverly to your emotional states. This is why hormones are so complicated; one sets another off, and so on. Therefore, understanding your own body's reaction to certain emotional situations is a good beginning.

One widely published method is to use positive self-talk and affirmations. Often, however, with severe emotional trauma positive conversation is not sufficient. *Whispering* represents a method of enhancing your own intuitive processes to provide self-feedback. This is combined with a proven and innovative exercise program. One component of the program includes reevaluating your own thinking processes about yourself. It is perhaps the hardest part.

Rejection

One related emotional trauma, for example, can be fear born from rejection. The reality of being rejected can happen to anyone at any stage in life. Rejection can include the emotional trauma involved in separation, divorce, or significant financial loss. This triggers fear based reaction throughout the body, causing severe stressors and resultant limbic actions. If there is a history of rejection experiences around previous hormonal peaks *(e.g., five years of age, teenage years)* then these reactions amplify. There is release of more and often uncontrolled chemical messengers to too many areas of the body.

In other words the stress is slower to recover from if you have suffered similar experiences when young. For example rejection sensations and self-blame while your parents were separating may trigger greater patterns of fright, flight or freeze reactions when this occurs to you personally. Especially, if you are already immune deficient or overly sensitive.

Keep in mind, however knowing this childhood history is only to assist your own confidence and understanding of what you are going through now. Your body is reacting to protect its own SEL, so admire it. So please do not overanalyze unremembered details from childhood, it is merely to help you understand the amount of pain, and the hypersensitivity in the neural receptors. Going over past events continually can lead to future problems in other hormonal receptors.

When the body cannot deal with the chemical messenger rush based on its previous preset balance one needs to be active fast. This condition can be altered mechanically through several approaches and when implemented soon enough avoids need for therapeutic counseling:

- Be positive about your own body
- Be involved in all manner of work or family holding self-belief in you and your positive role thereon
- Exercise, walk, but only at talk and walk speed for those who hate sport
- Work with others less fortunate than yourself, urgently volunteer when you feel sad, depressed or simply miserable
- Meet new friends, join toastmasters or speaking clubs, do humorous speeches

- Laugh, remember only what is important to your forward new lifestyle
- Be positive about your decisions regardless of what effect they have had, today is new
- Try continually to avoid negative people.

The way the body can interfere with its own good is fascinating, yet if we assume it is programmed at onset to achieve optimal balance it makes sense that an outpouring of a new positive emotive sensation can assist in resetting a new better balance. This can then simplify complex mental and emotional processes. Read the famous poem Desiderata again.

Emotional Trauma Does Not Imply Mental Weakness

The relationship between emotions and chemical messengers implies a relationship to the limbic system, glands, hormones, and related organs. It is not necessarily your conscious awareness of the emotional trauma that affects your pain; it is a result of chemical messenger releases affecting organs and tissue. It is organic in nature. There is a physiological response to all emotions. It is just not yet fully understood how far it affects other musculoskeletal injuries in midage people.

In your own social network; however, you may choose not to disclose a hormonal or stress involvement. For example, having a painful arm *from a torn rotator cuff* is certainly different to it being from *the divorce situation*. This simply reflects the high cultural value we place on sports and exercise. Sometimes, a mechanical cause of the trauma is needed psychologically, socially, and for your general well being.

Invest in your own self and begin describing your *trauma* in such a way that your own needs are constantly being met. For example, if sitting at a table full of sports people, talk about adhesions. It is not necessary to mention emotional trauma.

Emotional Stress and low anabolic steroid levels

One section of the adrenal axis (the A in LHPA) includes an array of hormones known to be associated with the adrenal gland. If the emotional trauma is producing ongoing stress or there is hypersensitivity to any stressor, there is an associated increase of *cortisol* with a consequential lowering of Dehydroepiandrosterone (*DHEA*).

Control the impact of stress and you must take more time for yourself, more than you could possibly perceive as being necessary. The importance of understanding the stressor is one way to achieve health. If the stressor is unknown and ongoing then the relationship between you and your *hormone whispering* is dysfunctional.

DHEA has a significant role related to estrogens and testosterone and boosts the immune system. The complexity of the relationship between this action and the thyroid glands is easily accessible on websites. Yet over-all if tiredness remains an ongoing symptom, and there are continued immune system problems (eg colds, undefined muscle aches) then consult your doctor for a thorough review. Consider any prescription suggestion of anabolic steroids (*short term DHEA replacement*) as wise. Six weeks maximum, review after 4 days without symptoms. Initiate again only after 4 sequential blood tests indicating low DHEA is ongoing, it is a complicated looping system and we do no harm to other hormones with these checks and balances.

What If My Life Is Always in Stress or Chaos?

Sorry. However, your hormones and neural pathways are affected by environmental factors whether you want to know it or not. Therapeutic interventions are not successful for capsulitis and frozen shoulders if your body is out of balance. Diet, life, love, and being liked are all part of that balance. Undo stress urgently, it is catastrophic. Standing your ground, believing in your own life journey is particularly important.

Identifying the Catalyst

The points below are to assist your *whispering*. Try to link ongoing or significant emotional trauma to the arm pain. The idea behind identifying something other than physical SEL is to see if the emotional trauma has impinged on your hormonal system in such a way that it has affected cortisol levels and therefore tissue strength, etc.

1. Identify the catalyst. What is the exact cause or stimulus that makes you feel helpless, sad, or overwhelmed, etc.?
2. Ask someone else how long ago it was that they saw you balanced, happy, and passionate.
3. Ask someone you trust if the same sad or bad event happened to him or her, what would he or she be doing *now?*

Activities to implement immediately:

- Do lots of things you love. This improves the oxytocin level, counteracting its nemesis cortisol.
- See yourself as better . . . more sexy . . . more clever . . . etc.
- Indulge in cuddles, hugs and random kind acts.
- Treat yourself to professional soft-tissue massages. These are excellent for improving local soft-tissue changes and secondary tightness.

Activities associated with pleasure, love, and inciting passion stimulate the mechanism involving hormone release and receptor balance. Happy hormones and active receptors are what you are trying to activate. The more people you have assisting your new positive thoughts, the better. Assist yourself more by asking at least three reliable friends to help, pray, or meditate for you.

Fear Is Another Indicator Things May Be Cortisol Charged

Fear affects hormones, hormones affects fascia. Fascia is a type of connective tissue. The fascia can be divided into three layers. The top layer is the superficial fascia, which is found immediately below the skin. The deep fascia follows this and then finally the subserous fascia, which is located deep within the body. It links through a complicated system and is directly affected by the emotions through the limbic system, polypeptides, and neurotransmitters. It is complex and beautiful, and functions optimally when balanced with low levels of stress hormones. Higher levels, especially for more than a few months, have roll-on health effects in every cell that the transmitting chemicals message.

Take care to invest in your own self after the diagnosis of a frozen shoulder. Searches on the Internet, other than this book, can be filled with doom and gloom. Avoid fear of the diagnosis, as this additionally affects your hormones. Use *hormone whispering* ASAP and frequently. Read on.

Acknowledging Emotional Factors and their relationship to hormone levels

Sometimes in giving your medical history you may mention an emotional trauma, but usually doctors are assessing musculoskeletal signs independently of anything else in your life.

A patient may simply be too shy to mention divorce, trauma in the family, or physical loss when consulting about shoulder pain. Some patients have reported to me having a suspicion that it was related, yet when they attempted to report it to the therapist, it was dismissed.

Pain can also be increased by emotional reactions unrelated to the injury per se. Fear causes certain chemical messengers to get involved in a bodily reaction. Each of these chemical messengers stays in the blood stream or target organs for different lengths of time. If there is a low-grade, ongoing emotional event or trauma, a lower-grade fear reaction sets the chemical messengers to use certain tissues to supply energy to either fight the fear or run away. For some reason your body stayed and froze. *Whispering* is a mental chance at reversing the fear, or at least minimizing the harm it has caused.

Another aspect of *hormone whispering* is gaining courage with your own *gut feel*. For example, if treatment progress is slower than it ought to be, try *whispering* for more clarity. It could be the current therapy approach is not right for your arm at this point in time. It does not make the therapy bad—just inappropriate now. It may involve your emotional trauma. This does not necessarily mean you need psychotherapy or even a counselor; try *whispering* initially as a way of dealing within to resolve solutions. Acknowledging that both physical and emotional factors may have contributed to the injury is the beginning of a good and much quicker healing phase. Please remember that if anyone has harmed you in love, you are not alone.

However, when we perceive something based on our own personal observation, due care has to be taken to see if that fits with important family and work colleagues' perceptions as well. To vary significantly is to be ostracized. This is fine if you are a leader or rebel or ready to leave, but if you are overweight, hitting an age milestone, or part of a cohesive team it can be incredibly difficult to move into newness alone.

One can even be ostracized when we try to fix something ourselves, or self-heal. The novelty of *hormone whispering* will make it unjustly judged in medical and therapy circles for a while, until at least they experience primary frozen shoulder themselves. Nonetheless you being effective and gaining positive control over your emotional SEL is difficult to measure by anyone else other than yourself. So remain positive, and sometimes we need reminders that we are progressing. Taking a measurement of pain and range of movement, or a photograph assists. The next chapter shows a few practical ways on how to assess simple shoulder movements.

CHAPTER 4

ASSESSING

Neuropeptides and their receptors are biological underpinnings of your awareness, manifesting themselves as emotions, beliefs, and expectations.
Dr. Candace Pert

Signals Needing Medical Consultation

There are some signals that indicate you should seek medical consultation:

1. Sleeping on that side causes *immediate* pain (eliminate fracture, tumor please)
2. The pain started with
   - a tumor (e.g., pituitary gland or after radiation)
   - a fall
   - a tear
3. You sustained an injury with force (e.g., sport injury, skiing, anything where the body propels forward of the shoulder at any angle). Some full-tendon thickness tears may require surgery, but not all. With full tendon tears, consider conservative measures only if it is the advice of a good surgeon. Age, external health, and both their and your attitude toward success will affect outcomes. Any avulsion from the bone *must* be treated urgently and may require surgical reattachment. Age matters.

Assessing Pain, Movement, and Emotional Strength

The three recommended assessments or outcome measures presented here are just a simplified way to provide you with quick feedback. Assessments are also useful tests for discovering more about your own arm pain or the effect of new movements or therapy success. Learn the following:

1. Pain—when still and when moving
2. Range of movement—three different ideas to test as a start
3. Emotional scoring—looking for things that are related to cortisol

> A Truth
> **Assessing for gain is no aim when no love remains.**

Where Is Your Pain?

On the body chart provided here, shade the areas where you experience pain.

Use either or both of the figures. Sometimes, one of the figures relates more to your sensations than the other.

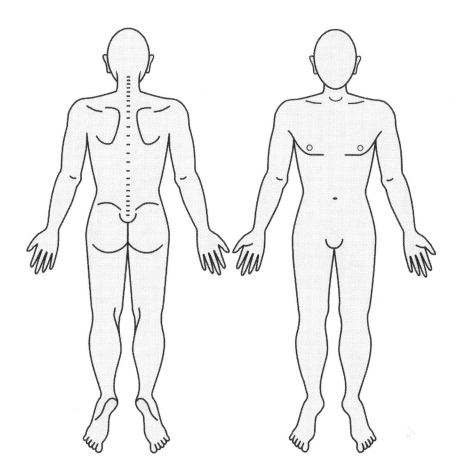

Scoring Pain on a Scale of 0 to 10

On a scale of 0 *(0/10 = no pain)* to 10 *(10/10 = extreme pain)*:

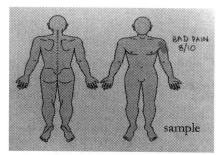

You can score pain for different situations:

Pain when you are resting (e.g., sitting upright and still)

Pain when it catches you (which movement?)

Mood-altering pain (optional)

Journal sample

Record scores to monitor progress. Sometimes, we may just need a physical reminder of how well we are doing. Don't bother if it is a hassle!

Date	*eg May 10th*	*eg May 16th*	
Pain resting	Average = 4/10		
Pain catching	Lifting handbag out of front seat of car = 8/10		
Mood-altering pain	Crankier than usual Less patient too		

Scoring Range of Movement

Select the three movements from the list below that affect you most. Test only once (e.g., before and once after a new exercise). Avoid repeating the testing movements over and over. Range will change daily, but overall movements must improve weekly to indicate you are on the right path; otherwise change repetitions, sequence or exercise strategies. Use a mobile phone, iPad, camera, etc., to record a picture of each movement or record the results in a diary or journal.

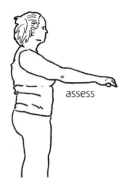

assess

Assess these movements

1. Measure your ability to brush your hair properly.
2. How high you can reach in your top/pantry shelf?
3. Cross your arms in front of your chest (under your breasts is best) and push slightly. (Be careful, because it can be painful.)
4. Reach behind your back, one hand at a time. How far up the back can you go? (Be careful, because it can be painful.). Often acute pain limits the movement to your side *eg no ability to touch bottom or back*. Measure it, and write it down or take a photo, it is important feedback.

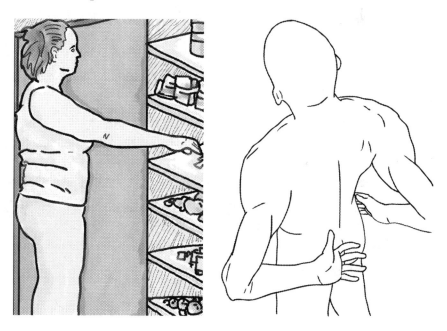

Journal sample

Date	May 10	
Brushing hair	Half range; could not lift shoulder up; had to bend **head** + pain 6/10	
Lifting arm	Got to chest height today	
Crossing arms	Unable to do push part of exercise + elbow stuck out	
Touching middle of back	Reached to my bottom only	

Use these assessments for your own evaluation. They are not important to retreat into or judge if you are a good *whisperer* or not.

Scoring Emotional Aspects

As I am proposing that an emotional element is probable in this injury we need to monitor and reassess something that you may be able to change without professional help. This focus is therefore on how you react to situations. For example:

1. Reactions to people who care
2. Reactions to others
3. Perception or judgment relating to the event or situation needing a solution and those involved
4. Degree of forgiveness to either yourself or others (e.g., "I forgive those who trespass or trespass against me")

Remember, pain itself can cause emotional responses, particularly if shoulder movement is required in your day-to-day activities. It can be incredibly frustrating and very painful. This can contribute to moodiness and inability to react well. Be kind to yourself.

Nonetheless, refusal to acknowledge an emotional trauma or a situation you are not acknowledging (or resolving) as a contributing factor may result in a longer recovery time. Ask for help as needed.

Calmly bring attention to any other potential symptoms:

- Are there other aspects of your life not making you happy?
- Are you so stressed you cannot make a simple decision?
- Are you often angry?
- Are you doing everything for others for receipt of love?
- Is there a trauma that really concerns you?
  - ➤ Will this take a long time to resolve?
  - ➤ If this trauma is behind you, are you still thinking about it *(looping)*?
- Is "it" helpless? "It" can be anything, anyone, any situation that takes unnecessary energy.
- Are you regularly negative about you?

Starting the Emotional Scoring

To start the emotional scoring ask yourself the following questions:

1. How much support for your injury, capsulitis, and/or pain are you getting—
   a. at work?
   b. at home?
   c. from loved ones?
2. How often do you *stand your ground*? (This means you have defended your own truth or belief (calmly) in any situation. Warning: do not stand your ground if it incites abuse. Seek professional help urgently.)

3. Is there something that you have to do that is stopping you from doing what you want to do?

These are the tasks that need focus to return hormonal output to a healing mode.

Journal sample

Date	May 10	Two weeks later
Support at work	Not relevant	Yes, boss says thank you every now and then.
Support at home	Sometimes	Sometimes, but I focus on doing it for me more often now & I can feel more contentment again . . . .
Supported with love	Not enough . . . aggressive teenager	I support myself more and leave the opinions of others as their own business. I was hurt by others' feelings more than I realized.
Stood my ground	Tend to give in to avoid conflict these days. Too tired to care, etc.	I asked my family to assist due to unfair workloads this week.

These journal entries simply reinforce behavioural changes we are making. They are not therapy nor should they isolate any single one of these behaviours as causal to the frozen shoulder.

CHAPTER 5

LEARNING TO WHISPER

Only those who attempt the absurd can achieve the impossible.
Albert Einstein

Whispering is something attainable by all. It is the start of moving health information forward from your unconscious SEL into the conscious mind without fear. For example, the ability to understand which direction a shoulder movement should take develops quickly with regular *whispering*. The goal is to ask your own body what its immediate needs are to heal.

Initially try and sit quietly in your own space. This should be a place where you are unlikely to be disturbed for at least fifty minutes. It is important to allow quiet time every day; it is a key to unlocking the emotional SEL's problems. Perhaps you need this more than you realize. You will actually eventually become more organized by taking this time.

Environment

Any learning process requires certain environments to optimize the chances of skill acquisition. *Whispering* is no different. Similar to meditation, this process of finding inner answers requires quiet, contemplative reflection time. Relax, recline, remain comfortable—it is not important to sit cross-legged. Any early random thoughts about family, work, etc., should be left aside, while your focus remains on the aspects of your SEL related to the shoulder condition.

Always light a candle (safely) within four yards of where you recline or lie. (Use of tea candles is best as they self-extinguish if forgotten.)

Should you hold lots of helplessness or intense sorrow within your emotional SEL, you may prefer a walking meditation instead. This may include walking or being close to trees and nature. The concept of altering hormones and other chemical messengers with gentle exercise and more positive self-talk is not new. *Whispering*, however, has to reach your emotional layer of SEL and alter its form; hence the need sometimes for long, hot showers postmeditation.

Questions to Start With

The use of visual, auditory, or sensory cues for hormone *whispering* is dependent on your own needs.

To start you off, try these questions and assume you are imagining a white screen in your mind (and behind your closed eyes). Ask your highest knowing:

- Is there a way to help?
  Did you see an answer on the screen or just know or hear a random thought or something else?
- Is there something I am not hearing or seeing?
  You may hear no, yes, or keep going or see a hint on that imaginary white screen. Your eyes may flick to things later to give you hints, so remember this question when in different rooms for best outcomes.
- Is there one way to cure these arm symptoms or is it many things?
  Many things need more direct asking; see below for some further information

Whispering is a skill anyone with enough time and self-respect can master. The best approach to *whispering* is the one that is most effective in altering your symptoms. Reread the parable (at the beginning of the book) just before you sit quietly, and the brain and higher consciousness can open out a little more to explore hidden streams. You may prefer to listen to the thoughts emerging rather than use screens or images.

Avoid skepticism and self-doubt. Be confident in your own self and take small steps to improve, remembering to remove fear. The key to successfully overcoming related emotional traumas and regaining hormonal balances in a safe and effective manner is to understand the importance of altering perceptions first.

Try *whispering* again and include the following request to your higher consciousness: How much of your arm pain is related to—

- not enough arm strength?
- an underlying hormonal imbalance?
- some combination of the above and an unresolved or recent emotional trauma?

While strengthening exercises are important, any emotional affects need to be explored initially or simultaneously. Here are a couple of questions that can lead to self-discovered emotional trauma:

- Have you suffered any severe emotional event in the last two to three years?
- What is the situation, event, or person that causes this severe emotional reaction?

Whispering

Whispering is you consciously guiding the unconscious on a journey for self-healing for the whole body. It is safe and self-paced. *Whispering*, per se, is the ability to link the needs of the emotional SEL to your symptoms, and then provide unique solutions back to your conscious mind to alter whatever is needed. Often this causes perceptions and self-talk to change, too.

Try a simple question over and over: *why* . . .
Not when, not how, just why.
Why have I got this reaction to my . . .
Why do I become overly emotional every time someone . . .
Why am I sore?

Avoid having no confidence in your ability to hear, feel, or see answers. Some say that *hormone whispering* is similar to heightening the internal intuition. Stay quiet for ten to thirty minutes after an intense questioning of your usual reactions. Write down random thoughts. Avoid denying answers. Let them sit without solution, as it is still a start and perhaps all the body needs to hear.

One has to have enough self-love to heal this. Avoid launching into too many questions, justifications, guilt trips, or overreacting to answers you instinctively know. These habits shut *whispering* down. The body fights itself. If your health is being affected, the *whispering* heightens not only awareness of that, but advanced *whispering* may even offer solutions. However, what if that solution is something big you need to change? Then discuss it with a trusted friend to see if they agree with your new perception. Is there something in your life that is too stressful or demanding—too much work and not enough pay or praise? Your *whispering* will heighten this awareness as long as you are prepared for solutions; until then it may just decide to keep the current pain or loss of movement.

Avoid any solution that harms more. I advise, due to the potential strength of the feedback loop, caution with sudden desires to alter relationships, family processes, and friendships. Take your time and plan wisely; open love out. If it means you downsize, then do it with gusto, imagining yourself better off in the end. If it means you are fat, forty plus, and lazy, embrace it and be sexy in that skin. The reason the body acts crazy is you are not hearing what it really wants. Inside you is a mechanism to be happy and healthy. Also allow your spirit to be *"at peace with God, whatever you conceive Him to be, and whatever your labors and aspirations, in the noisy confusion of life keep peace with your soul"* (from Max Ehrmann's poem *Desiderata*).

Alternative to that but not as strong is to just keep faking contentedness in all aspects of your life until you get enough hormones on your side, then gain strength using the 5 x 5 exercise (see chapter 8). Trust enough to know the *whisper* will alter something within, and your body will at some point know how to do it another way.

Whispering is not necessarily easy to develop for those who are not as sensitive; however, the feeling of getting a few pieces of information validated with outcome assessments can strengthen your *whispering* confidence significantly.

Whispering to Heal the Emotional SEL

To assist in the *whispering* process for resolutions in the emotional SEL you have to understand how to initially disassociate from the event that causes the trauma. Remember the mud in the parable. Any shoulder signs and symptoms need to be ignored for a short time while you concentrate on the body's feelings, emotional reactions, or *stagnating emotional SEL energy*.

Can you separate the actual event from the way you respond or react to it? If not you need help from a professional or should attend a great healer who can move outside energy layers around to benefit your physical SEL's perception without repeating the trauma.

The body can heal itself to a certain level and then wait. The waiting or receiving of pain elsewhere perhaps makes one reflective of work or situations were other unhappiness lies.

Tragedy on a scale of many losses can cause all parts of the organic system to malfunction, but no matter how fit and sporty you are, the important thing is to try to accept other invisible energy blocks as currently in the way of healing your shoulder, indigestion, or chest pain.

If your brain has selected a negative pathway and keeps looping back and forth ask a friend for a new perspective, please. Take the most positive person's opinion to be your new start. Reflect on your personal reactions rather than the actual event. You can change the perspective, and then your reactions, but you can't undo time or the situation that has been. Forgive yourself first and foremost. It remains important for your own health to be less defensive, less judgmental, and open to new reactions to what was undoubtedly a bad thing. If you are understanding enough of that process, further change in the emotional SEL will occur with *whispering.*

Again forgive your early responses, as you have done the best you can to date. Some feel rejection and respond with distrust in an ongoing way. Resentment, crying, dismissal, and even eating chocolate can be past reactions that need to change. Another defensive response is to place blame. For example, some take all who had a hand in the event and blame them, while others overly blame themselves. Most of these types of reactions also emit from an underlying fear. Whisper to find out what your fear really is about.

Whispering and Pain

Pain is within your personal control. You can take drugs to medicate and dull it, and then try and use that time to heal. To medicate as a sole solution is another matter.

Whispering to assist your pain acts in two ways:

1. By altering perception of how to do movements through learning to trust and return control to your own consciousness.
2. By altering your reactions to emotional events that spark hormonal and neurochemical firing that cause hypersensitivity in the pain pathways. Even though some methods of therapy include allowing permission to rebel or be angry or defensive, if you walk away from that event with elements of fear and

associated reactions (please note that feeling rejected is fear based) then the pain remains. Therefore the *whispering* when focused can further clarify ways to—

- alter your response;
- vary your exposure to that emotional trauma and avoid any similar situation;
- avoid reacting to other people;
- protect your own SEL (a body in danger should be allowed to tap into its gut feeling anywhere, anytime).

During *whispering* times some thoughts, images, or even body sensations may pop fleetingly—for example, the fact that your body alters its position repeatedly, or the body feels certain sensations warning you not to be around a person or situation. If emotional SEL releasing starts with sensations of anger, resentment, etc., please remain in your private space. Learn to trust your body's process of release without going through old emotional pathways. Often lighting a candle during the process and following through by jumping into a shower afterwards for a sense of release and washing the old stuff away assists. Repeat it over and over until you feel a difference in pain. Repeating strong sensations of anger may indicate your body requesting assistance from higher help. Be that prayer, requests for family interventions, or even cognitive behavioral therapies, your *whispering* when achieved optimally will guide you. Ask, pause, and then whisper *for your greatest good* before entering the fray.

"The thought popped into my head that there is a reason this occurred. It did not seem far. I was being criticized for something I had not done again. Two people joined in. I started my usual way of defending and rationalizing their view; they were senior to me, and I had to take care. Then I whispered for my greatest good. A sense of calm came over me, and I was distracted with another thought for a second; this mellowed my emotion to some degree. It enabled me to stay quiet long enough to gather strength within my own SEL. Unfair situation, but not worth aggression. There and then my belief in me had to be greater than their collective opinions. It was hard, as I was

usually flexible and giving, kind rather than internally strong. I whispered over and over again—stay quiet, speak your truth calmly and quietly after they have exhausted their opinions. The shoulder did not spasm as much as usual either as I remained in my own power so to speak."—Claire

---

A Truth
Pain attributed to another person is a strange attitude to take. That person, after all, is not feeling it.

Q & A

Will my capsulitis really take two to three years to recover?

Yes, if the neural transmitters and emotional SEL remain altered. The body can take that long to learn how to adjust to the malfunction. Hormones reset balances even when there are ongoing higher outputs. This is not necessarily healthy for all organs. That is why *whispering* brings the attention back to emotional trauma and specifically works to alter the reaction and continuing fear-based behaviors. Whisper, work it out, and recovery will be more immediate.

One question I ask my patients is WHY they have the frozen shoulder. Whisper over and over until you are clear on this. This is very separate to when, how, or what. So: Not when did you get it. Not how did you get it. Not even what tissue or tendon it is. *Why?*

When the body understands you are calling it forward to ask it to provide answers via thoughts, sensations, dreams, or symbols, it will naturally work towards homeostasis faster. But can you decipher the clues? For example, sometimes your eyes may glance at furniture (e.g., a chair to rest in), photos, family faces, or the site of an old remembered event to prompt change in you. These are clues to needs; endeavor to decipher them during quiet time or meditations.

This condition can heal itself over a one year period if you are diligent with exercises and maintain a positive mental attitude. You can speed that up further with *whispering*. Remember that the actual shoulder tissue itself heals very fast; the other systems depend on active participation and your ongoing reactions, habits, and perceptions.

What interferes with whispering?*

- Fear, especially fear that you are not able to do it, is a huge factor leading to interference. Let yourself be open to being as intuitive as anyone else for a short time, and magic happens.
- Skeptics—they bring the entire world to a grinding halt.

What does "self-heal" mean?

Simple: you are involved in the therapy. You guide and decide by internal consultations, for example, using *whispering* or meditation. There are many self-healing techniques in existence. Please choose the one most efficient for you.

---

* *Clients reading the parable often note they think of different reasons for the outpouring of emotions each time. It can be used as a starting point for overlooked causes of the current arm pain and frozen shoulder. Refer to the parable over and over if stuck. Strong whisperers experience sensations that alter movements automatically again before onset of symptoms. Not knowing what movement to do at any given time is an example of an unlinked body or, according to the parable, blocked and muddy tributaries. Random thoughts may start the process and form another way of knowing what you need to change. These sensations may even feel like they are coming from high above. Be confident with yourself again, develop a system of cognitive awareness, and watch your life change. The trust takes time to develop again between the unconscious and conscious after a significant emotional event. Even outcome measures that may seem trivial or silly to you are necessary early on to heighten your attention on your own ability to succeed in your own self. This strengthened core is the start of your own human ability, or self-developed consciousness, to deal with your own body's indispositions. It takes time.*

What if I think it is my rotator cuff or tendonitis?

Emotional states are rarely discussed at physical therapy appointments, yet it is widely acknowledged that the performance of elite athletes is affected by emotions and mental state. Why, therefore, should this be overlooked in dealing with your condition? If you work towards actively using a positive mental attitude as part of your program, then you are beginning the self-healing process, no matter what the cause of the trauma is. *Whispering* works with or without there being an underlying emotional trauma. It is solid.

"I tried the exercise the physical therapist gave me three times before I threw the tape/elastic away. It hurt more afterwards, and the concept of "no pain no gain" for me was not right. After reading your work, I listened to my own shoulder . . . . The movement was actually similar to one in the back of your new manuscript, so I thought I should tell others that I never believed in myself enough to think my body could guide me to a movement better than someone trained, but it did. I actually told my therapist I did her exercises, and she was so proud how well they worked . . . . Oops—as secretly I did my own! Will have to stand my ground more though won't I. Thanks."—G.

Your emotional SEL will and does interferes with physical SEL. *Whispering* assists sorting it out. This can be done simultaneously with any therapeutic intervention. It need not be spoken of to the therapist.

Medical practitioners and surgeons want their procedures to be successful for the patients that come to them. If you are able to work on the emotional aspects before committing the time and money to their practice, results are bound to be better. Allow enough time to resolve as much as possible yourself. In fact, you may just resolve the condition on your own in record speed.

A One-to-One Experience with a Therapist
Using Hormone Whispering

Patient: *(clarifying the process) Are you saying what makes me upset makes my shoulder pain?*

Therapist: *Yes, and more. What are the biggest things that make your grief?* *(Note the term* pain *is not mentioned)*

Patient: *That I cannot dress myself without pain. That I cannot lift my arm to do housework or work. My sore arm makes me feel old, unfit, and fat. (long pause) My relationship with my husband.*

Therapist: *Thinking more on the last two reasons as specific contributing factors to the condition, do you think getting an operation will change that?*

Patient: *(laughs) Only if it is to surgically remove fat and improve tone.*

Therapist: *Laughing is good, yet I want to ask about the relationship with your husband: is there fear involved? (The talk evolved into counseling to focus attention on how to stop reacting to certain home situations. In this case there was no abuse, only trust problems that linked into a feeling of being abandoned, etc.)*

CHAPTER 6

COMMON QUESTIONS ABOUT SHOULDERS AND WHISPERING

Forgiveness is letting go of the hope that the past can be changed.
Oprah Winfrey

It is the premise of this book that chemical messengers link the emotional to the physical. The actions of one system are integrated and in this case harm the other; reversing this for the action of healing requires focused self-appraisal. It has to become a habit to outthink the abnormal functions within a damaged system. Hence the *whispering*. The *hormone whispering* affects emotional SEL. Emotional SEL can also be quickly healed with biofield therapies (e.g., Therapeutic Touch™). Nonetheless, you should accept responsibility for your own emotional reactions as soon as possible. Enjoying a healing session, thinking positively about it and the practitioner, and then choosing the correct exercise routine (described in Chapter 7/8) will make it a far more efficient and longer-lasting healing. Do not do it unless you are ready to accept that something has to be released, forgiven, or denied.

The linking is not only through the hormones and their target organs; it involves polypeptides and neurochemicals and other forces that simply are not visible yet. It affects billions of cells in your body at any one time. Additionally, *hormone whispering* tempers movement, therapy, and exercises to appropriate levels for your condition at any stage. Having someone else move off the emotional bad SEL is a great idea, but take care to find the best healer.

Menopause, Hormones, and Middle Age

It is probable that age-related hormonal changes are occurring in the body of a menopausal female, which can additionally weaken the mechanisms usually in place to protect the body from low-grade stressors. The relevance of physical catabolic-based injuries to preexisting hormonal *disbalances* is a new field. If frozen shoulder, as cited in scientific journals, is more common in women over forty-five years of age, then what specifically connects this condition to female menopause? Could it be that excess cortisol, acting to weaken tissue, specifically creates a little drop in the shoulder ball-and-socket joint secondary to capsule degradation? Or is one simply more prone to emotional highs and lows? Have we *learned reactions* more prone to draining weakened corticosteroid loops? Have receptor sites altered? Or have old neural pathways perhaps opened to misrepresentation in the current event? Is our perception, tolerance, or acceptance varied with age, thereby altering chemical discharge?

The body, in all its absolute brilliance, reacts to pull the joint back into itself. We call it capsular adhesions and inflammation and think it is bad. I think it is brilliant.

Are You a Little Slack with Your Exercise Program for the Upper Body?

If you put everyone else before yourself, including work, home, and family, your exercise and walking routine may be neglected. Sometimes, worrying about it can add even more stress or guilt and result in higher levels of stress chemical agents.

You may feel that trying to fit one more thing into your day, no matter how good it might be for you, would be the last straw. This indicates significant involvement of emotional SEL. Go and get healings or therapeutic massage (gentle touch) as soon as possible.

Do You Have a Flattening of the Muscles in the Deltoid Area?

The optimal shape of the deltoid muscle is rounded, and the only indent is where the insertion meets the bone of the upper arm, see picture A below. It should be a rounded muscle.

Look at your affected arm in the mirror. Compare it to the other arm. If it is flat, or indents near the top of the arm, it means you are already too weak. The shoulder has to be strengthened (even with the use of painkillers) as soon as possible. Can you achieve the 5 x 5 series in Chapter 8 yet? This phase requires *whispering* with *Shoulder CPR* exercises first (refer to chapter 7). If you manage to enhance your own control and keep the joint in its socket before any other movement, further injury can be prevented.

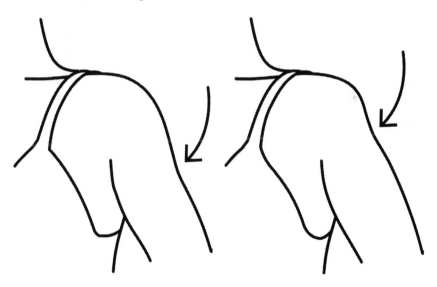

The reversal of this laxity is critical to preventing the freezing stage if it has not already started. Sometimes, the related pain can be described as a pulling pain or intermittent irritation. It can also be (misleadingly) tender in specific tendons or junctions. Refer to commonly labeled areas in the rotator cuff illustration.

Deltoid insertion

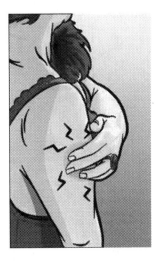

The deltoid insertion is the lowest point where the deltoid muscle, the thick, triangular muscle covering the shoulder joint, attaches to bone. Pain at this location is secondary to lean muscle mass wasting; it may even feel warm and spongy if you touch directly on the deltoid insertion point. The small, circular inflammation is a sign that the muscles have weakened to such a point that overuse syndrome has begun at the insertion of this muscle; perhaps even connective tissue is breaking down. It remains tender for a few days only. I am unsure as to the reason for its presence, but it is a common precursor to range of movement loss. This phase requires *whispering* with the *Shoulder CPR* exercises urgently and repeatedly, then exercising passively through available movement (refer to chapter 7). Preventing the adhesive capsulitis at this point is the best outcome you are going to get. Move onto the 5 x 5 series (chapter 8) as soon as possible after warmth in the tissue resolves.

Is Your Movement Already Limited?

The freezing stage of capsulitis is when the movement decreases. Lifting the arm outwards is particularly hard.

Remind yourself to push the joint into the socket to prevent excess adhesions, capsular thickening, and vascularization.

The emotional trauma should be also resolved to reverse, as possible, the chemical messenger patterns causing the cellular weakness. For example, side effects of some messengers can weaken and loosen tissues in the shoulder. Annoying the limbic system with more reactions is the worst thing you can do. Eliminate all fear and trauma. This phase requires *whispering* with the *Shoulder CPR* exercises urgently and repeatedly, then the froggy-flop series as soon as possible to avoid complications in the low back, cervical areas and other shoulder. Avoid excess fear. This exercise (Froggy series) can seem impossible but ends up one of the more effective moves you can ever do for your long term flexibility and arm. Preventing the adhesive capsulitis at this point is the best outcome you are going to get. Move onto the 5 x 5 series (chapter 8) as soon as possible after warmth in the limbic tissue resolves.

What Is the Rotator Cuff?

The rotator cuff is made up of a small group of muscles and tendons that hold the shoulder stable in its joint. Refer to the illustration for a guide: if you palpate your own shoulder area, you may be able to feel a specific ridge that relates to certain tendons. It can be very locally painful to feel. Physical therapists know the exact spot for each of these tendons. (Ouch!) A diagnosis of a *rotator cuff injury* can be made from this palpation. However, inflammation of surrounding supporting tissue or the onset of capsulitis is going to make a lot of nearby tissue sensitive. When there is strong finger pressure and affected lymph tissue in the same spot, you may erroneously be diagnosed with a rotator cuff injury. The process of healing then is in the hands of the practitioner, who may never consider discussing your related social and emotional history. Also, scans cannot always eliminate the surrounding tissue areas, particularly the involvement of limbic and support tissue. I propose that tendon palpation independent of thorough medical and social history does not take into account capsule and connective tissue irritation from metabolic changes.

Additionally, when you attend some medical practitioners or therapists who are strong in their own personal belief systems, their understanding about mechanisms of injury may get in the way of a successful outcome for you. Don't waste money. Use *whispering* to get a clear answer about your prognosis with their style.

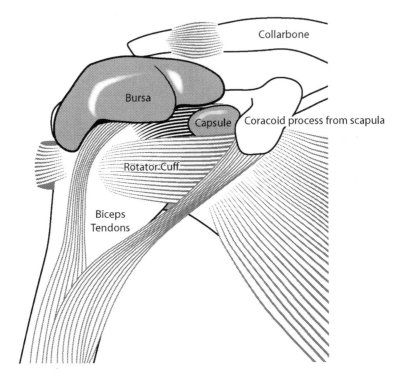

Biceps tendons are two long, thin tendons that extend from the biceps muscle to the top of the shoulder socket (see the illustration). Localized pain along either tendon is usually associated with a physical trauma. Often you can localize a single tender point. It is not hormonally related unless other areas are tender or inflammatory markers are high. Trauma or tears can be easily diagnosed by a scan. Ensure, however, that any tear revealed relates to original trauma, on overextension with exertion in direction of biceps action. Additional to the tear may be an underlying *disbalance* in joint mechanics. Take into account also any prior or subsequent emotional traumas that may complicate an otherwise standard tissue-healing time.

A classic injury scenario is reaching from the front seat of a car to the backseat to lift a briefcase or handbag. This injury should, however, resolve with due care. Avoid repeating aggravating angles for at least six to eight weeks after the original injury and avoid pre-tear patterns of movement.

Bursitis or Capsulitis?

Capsulitis is inflammation of capsular tissue. This is usually between joint surfaces. *Adhesive capsulitis* is synonymous with the term *frozen shoulder*, but loosely includes closely related connective tissue.

Bursitis, on the other hand, is an inflammation in a bursa, or fluid-encased sac supporting easy glide movements. Bursae sit over joint areas where they can serve to counter high friction. Getting optimum benefit from a bursa encompasses knowing how to keep the area balanced from each possible movement direction. Lack of strength in any direction, poor postural habits, and overuse tend to slide a tendon off its optimal track.

Is a tender bursa area therefore a result of *disbalance* or subtle separation of the ball-and-socket joint? In athletes overuse tenderness is a different mechanism to the drop in shoulder-joint position stemming from menopause or emotional trauma. More research is required. Nonetheless, tenderness in the bursa is easily diagnosed by specialist physical therapists.

Bursitis in isolation would imply an unusual injury, or more likely an overuse, singular, directional injury. It involves rotational sequences and joint dysfunction. So again, it is impossible to have a local inflammation without some disarray of functioning joint surfaces. Therefore try the same exercises, apply due diligence, and self-assess. Alternatively isolating the problem to one area is problematic if no one guides you in repair. If, for example, you are having therapy/steroid injections (which can work in bursitis), can you still *please* discover the cause? If you are diagnosed with an impingement injury, do you think it was sport related? A traditional impingement of physical tissue (e.g., from sport) may require retraining in some very basic movement functions and roller exercises (refer to chapter 7).

Do You Hear Cracks, Grating, and Clunks with Movements?

Try and evaluate each sound, as some cracks are OK but others not. Some people can be scared by having these noises; others enjoy them while believing it is a sign of more movement. Hormone whisperers will follow their instincts and avoid sounds that appear to be aggravating symptoms and enjoy crunching as range of movement or quality of movement improves. Monitor this using your range of movement assessments for reassurance.

What about Medical Interventions?

Whisper and meditate, who would know more about your shoulder: a specialist, a chiropractor, a surgeon, or you? Perhaps they will know more about the condition and anatomy; however, you may know more about underlying causes that will affect outcome. Whisper and meditate to discover who you need to work with to cure your pain. Other related conditions may need other specialists involved in the future.

Believing that you can self-heal is one thing, but believing that your surgeon can operate successfully is another. The concept of believing you are going to get better is incredibly important to the healing process. If you need a surgical procedure, please be sure you have resolved all emotional traumas. Additional surgical intervention that provokes fear will only exacerbate something.

For those undertaking any interventions, remember to slow down, ask your body to assist the procedure, and listen to professional advice with caution. I have seen far too many given *permission* to return to sport too soon and reinjure later. For example, do not lift, carry, or twist, no matter how "great" you feel, for a few weeks. (Read through the exercises in chapters 7 and 8 and chapter 9 about return to sport.)

Keep in mind that it is unlikely that a specialist sports surgeon will be interested in your relationship issues or other emotional traumas. He or she will focus on the shoulder condition as it presents. Be careful, therefore, to share the symptoms that will encourage the practitioner to act with diligence and accuracy.

Some tests include pain scales, shoulder range of movement in all directions, and even holding your arms out sideways against force. These tests can aggravate, however they are considered important to diagnose ruptures and the tendons involved. **Be very specific if pain is the same or more intense in any single direction.** Do not try to pre-empt the professional: remain honest, succinct and accurate. Surgeons have limited time. Consider what pain you have in what situations before the consultation *eg diffuse pain over all areas . . . . is a different diagnosis to pre freezing stages when sudden acute pain stabs and this impacts on surgical outcomes, good surgeons want to decipher this detail for success.*

You may also be asked what angles of movement create most difficulty and which specific tasks. They diagnose fast, be accurate please. Rehearse all beforehand including aggravating movements, angles and pain scales at night. Talk about your experiences of stress briefly. Ask should you be on anabolic steroids. Stress takes away the body's ability to create sufficient hormone *(eg DHEA)* in some people, anabolic steroids in short term prescriptions is worthy of a trial with therapeutic interventions prior to surgical chaos.

Energy treatments like the one below is unlikely to be a surgeon's flavor, yet moderate evidence exists for its effectiveness on tissue in vivo and vitro. This is part of the new paradigm for shifting the emotional component of *primary frozen shoulder.* It will assist pre freeze and in total prevention of secondary tightnesses longer term.

What is Biofield Energy treatment?

This is a method of using energy, chi, prana, or universal energy to work around the body. Many techniques promote alterations in mood, ability to gain relaxation and solve unconscious emotional problems. Yet all therapy needs to have you as the center, it needs to be done with the intent of power from within you rather than the practitioner's force. This is the safest way.

I am most familiar with Therapeutic Touch™ due to its intent of *the greatest good*. Therapeutic Touch™ (TT) is a technique developed by Dora Kunz and Dr. Dolores Kreiger, the former a gifted healer and the latter a registered nurse and educator. The technique has a more rigorous teaching and mentoring approach than most biofield energy techniques and is certified through the Therapeutic Touch International Association. I invested a number of years in this process myself. The major subtle energy that TT engages is *prana,* or life energy, with the key being the intentionality of the practitioner.[*]

TT is perhaps the most researched of the healing methods, having been investigated under controlled studies exploring and demonstrating its effectiveness in relaxation, wound healing, and bone synthesis.[**] Additionally, as evaluated by the McGill Melzack Pain Questionnaire, TT has been shown to be effective in relieving tension headaches and pain.[***] Turner et al. reported a positive effect on burn patients and proposed that TT reduces anxiety and may decrease pain perception and enhance immune function.[****]

These reports have been criticized as insignificant because they did not employ rigorous double-blind trials. However, in a world-class study and a brilliant effort to determine if TT actually works at a cellular level, experimenters removed bone tissue, amalgamated it

---

[*] *What is spirit? What is Healer?* By Krieger. Nurse healers Professional associates International Conference, Wainright House, Rye, NY. 2000.

[**] *Healing Research, Volume II. Consciousness, Bioenergy and Healing* (Vol. II). Medford, NJ, USA: Wholistic Healing Publications. Benor. 2004: 332.

[***] *Effects of Therapeutic Touch on Tension Headache Pain,* by E. Keller and V. M. Bzdek. *Nursing Research* 35 (2), 1986: 101-6

[****] *The Effect of Therapeutic Touch on Pain and Anxiety in Burn Patients,* by J. G. Turner, A. J. Clark, D. K. Gauthier, and M. Williams. *Journal of Advanced Nursing* 28 (1), 1998: 10-20

with preparations in such a way as to isolate osteoblasts, then had TT healers use TT over the plastic culture dishes, thus eliminating the factors of a patient's opinion, intent, or belief.* Measurements were made of osteoblast synthesis and mineralization. This rigorously controlled in vitro study of osteoblast cultures (that is, preparations made from the bone chips of patients) demonstrated that TT could alter DNA synthesis, differentiation, and mineralization in healthy bone with four 10-minute treatments over a period of two weeks. The same study also found a significant alteration of messenger RNA expression for Type-I collagen, bone sialoprotein, and alkaline phosphatase, recording a decrease of these markers in culture dishes with an osteosarcoma-derived cell line. (Osteosarcoma is a cancer of the bone, and these cell lines are developed specifically for experimentation.) In a personal communication from one of the TT therapists taking part in the study, she reported the publishing journal's close scrutiny of the tabled results and the surprise of one of the researchers at the positive outcomes.** Perhaps TT and its use of energy is simply too at variance for Western medicine to collate as useful.

While other energy healing practices such as Qi-gong, Reiki, and Healing Touch also may position their hands four to eight inches away from the body the effect does vary with practitioner and setting, as does the intent and natural energy output. **I recommend four to seven TT sessions with a qualified practitioner, especially for the painful *menopausal*-related frozen shoulder.** My personal belief is that *hormone whispering* should guide the sessions—that is; who, when and where. But this therapy is novel for most people, hence the guideline. A sense of relaxation is normal; often memory *fuzziness* is a good sign if you relax into it and sleep that night without stress. However, when asking anything, please ensure that the practitioner's

---

Therapeutic Touch Affects DNA Synthesis and Mineralization of Human Osteoblasts in Culture, by A. Jhaveri, S. J. Walsh, Y. Wang, M. McCarthy, and G. Gronowicz. *Journal of Orthopaedic Research* 28 (11), 2008: 1541-46

positive intent remains *"for the greatest good"* at all times; when consulting a practitioner for a musculoskeletal disorder, treatment intent may be directed at pain or stiffness instead of the greatest good, thereby potentially bypassing the very method able to stimulate hormonal changes required.

Other Questions Worth Whispering About Before Consultations

Should I try a second cortisone injection?

The answer to this will vary depending on the history. *Whispering* and meditation is important to determine your own responses. The following questions may prompt your intuition a little more. Did you try other measures first? Have you been applying all the strategies in this book? Have you kept up the 5 x 5 exercises (they really do work) and FroggyFlop long enough? Then, if after all that intervention you have no emotional trauma, go to a shoulder specialist knowing you have done your best and you are mentally prepared for his or her opinions.

What if I disagree (or have a gut feeling) that the doctor's exercise is not right for me?

Then do not do it. *Hormone whispering* will assist these dilemmas. Use this book's exercises for a start to a new way (see chapter 7) for a few days, and you will have a comparative approach to gather strength in your own ability to chose solutions. Remember to use the assessment movements before and after new regimes for optimum guidance.

Can I ask you to assist?

Yes. It works like a distant healing link. If you are more into technology there will be an author webpage and YouTube links. However, the energetic link via God is far more potent, regardless of belief.

CHAPTER 7

EXERCISES USING WHISPERING

We are what we repeatedly do. Excellence,
then, is not an act, but a habit.
Will Durant

Exercising the shoulder is important and not negotiable. Muscular tone is required to maintain the ball *in* the shoulder joint socket. Strength has to be regained from any catabolic steroid effects as soon as possible. Intermittent shoulder discomfort, a nagging twinge, or a spontaneous need to massage areas of the arm and neck is a signal to alter:

- Positions (more than one joint)
- Strength
- Joint *disbalance*

While a few of the exercises in this book complete all three requirements simply and efficiently, the Shoulder CPR is an easy start. No matter how high you lift the shoulder it can be started gently. Read the Shoulder CPR instructions carefully first, and remember to measure range of movement before and after. Easy-to-use exercises like this done throughout your day PREVENT frozen shoulder. It is very, very successful.

Exercise in functional, preferably familiar directions, and do exercises you like. Make them up if you don't like these. However, my personal preference is to avoid isolating single muscles (although this is commonly prescribed) as it does not imitate your real-life ability.

Each time a direction or movement hurts, try *whispering*, and use the pain positively as a way of improving your method. Each exercise needs variation in movement style, repetitions, and starting position, and the *hormone whispering* can guide that.

Whispering and Safety

If you are truly monitoring your own body, then the knowledge of when to start and stop is clear. *Whispering* is important; override any of the book's instructions if you feel, sense, or hear that a particular movement or exercise is not right. **Never force pain**.

If you are attempting a new movement direction, please use gentle movements—slow and steady with as much pleasure as possible.

If it catches or causes pain: Stop, Breathe, and Decide

- Is it my body saying, "No way. Stop"?
  guide: Then stop.
- Is it my body reminding me that there is something I have forgotten, am not doing, or am not saying?
  guide: Guide the arm more slowly; be sure to test the movement before and after. Then if still feeling pain from the exercise, move to another one or more Shoulder CPR. Ask your deep self to assist; it may be that more emotional work needs doing first. Perhaps leave it for a week and then retry while whispering.
- Is it my conditioned fear? Is the body stopping itself out of habit?
  guide: Trying it gently while breathing in and out and smiling assists. Reward yourself mentally; for example, say out loud, "That was easier than I expected." Repeat a second time more slowly. Try another repetition without moving to full possible range. If you have tried twice gently and it is worse, then that exercise is not correct: simply stop. Normal levels of pain return shortly after any experimentation. Keep having a go.

Meditation Can Also Form Part of an Efficient Whispering and Exercise Program

Meditation can be useful for the frontal cortex and therefore related neural and chemical pathways. Meditation is not *whispering*, although *hormone whispering* attacks beliefs and bad perceptions the meditative state precludes conscious awareness thereof.

One needs to be very comfortable. Try to semirecline rather than lie down flat or sit up rigidly cross-legged. You need to find your own best place and position, somewhere quiet.

One of the reasons mental attitude is so important is to activate your own belief system in your own ability to fix parts that are yours. Meditation can heighten your own ability to hear the specific needs for frozen shoulder. Initially however this requires you to embrace two points:

- Accept that you can alter behavior by using your own *power of the mind.*
- Take time and patiently calm any erroneous or negative self-talk.

Once you have a handle on these, try to recline for ten to twenty minutes and discipline yourself to ask for the greatest good in this moment in time. One favorite is to ask the following:

"Body, I love you. How can we work together so that happiness and health is the new way? I know it can be with less guilt or pressure, as my hormones are renewing and I want the greatest good there is!"

Close your eyes; the sequence usually is that your brain will automatically leak things it has to remember first. There is really no need to urgently write it all down or panic about remembering. Relax into the calm as the brain settles into a slower pattern; it may have just needed to push those messages at you first. Anxiety about memory needs to be set aside.

Next stage is a much needed little rest; you may even get some ideas and then doze—doze and then wake up clearer and more happy than when you started. Sometimes people recall nothing at all following this phase. If your body decides to keep the consciousness out of the healing time, then understand that this slight rest and slowing of brain activity allows for self-readjustments internally anyway. Some people may adjust their workday slightly or naturally sit or position themselves differently after a session. Do not be alarmed if you go into a deep trance and then dream a little, as this is another way the body's unconscious SEL will talk to your emotional body from time to time. There is no need to understand it all in detail. Your body may not even want conscious thought patterns interrupting its own healing time.

If this is properly conducted, eventually you will wake up and should feel bright and light. The best thing to do next is to go outdoors and have a short, brisk walk. It clears the mind even more. If you are able to, do a two-minute jog to start the 5 x 5 series. During this burst of activity after meditation it can become very clear what it is that you will be doing next as thoughts and determination are given a new lease on life.

In total, these twenty minutes will increase the efficiency of your day in a stabilized, less emotive way.

Your work can become more efficient, and you should use the *hormone whispering* to adapt to your situation (e.g., apply during a lunch break—efficiency is a result). Even which exercise to begin with can be revealed.

Shoulder Circles

This is an old and traditional yet very effective exercise.

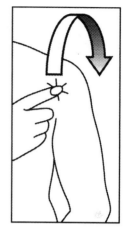

In any position, move the whole shoulder, circling *backward,* without lifting the elbow out or moving your forearm much. Focus on shoulder blade circling. Experiment with positioning your fingers gently on different points of the shoulder area while circling for a more advanced effect.

Tips

Repeat smoothly as often as you feel is right. For example, try ten to thirty at a time. It usually feels more effective for participants who get tight in their back and neck muscles as a result of the painful arm.

This exercise has been around for a very long time and is generally undervalued because of its simplicity. Use it wisely; assess it based on comfort of the area rather than range of movement.

Another variation worth considering is to use a tiny, very soft ball in the back of an office chair at your preferred point and explore with *whispering* how many shoulder circle repetitions you need to help the discomfort. (Note: too many or too large a ball can hurt.)

"The difference this makes to the tightness in my neck during the workday is extraordinary . . . . I am expert on how to place my finger in the exact sore spot to maximize the effect. My shoulder blades sit more evenly now too . . . . So easy, thank you."—Paul

Passive Arm Lifts

Lift your painful shoulder without moving any arm muscles on that side. Use the opposite hand. This is a passive movement as the good arm totally takes the weight of the sore arm. Prevent any contraction while lowering the arm. Any twitch of activity may cause pain, so take care while learning this exercise; it is difficult to achieve full passivity.

In the shower

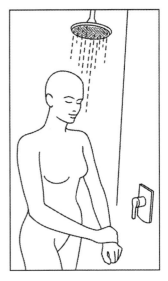

Grasp the wrist firmly with your other hand and take the sore shoulder for a smooth, slow ride, in any direction that feels comfortable. It need not be far. Usually forward is easier than sideways. But accidentally using the muscles around the shoulder can be enough to bring tears to your eyes, so keep a passive hold! Often, only thirty seconds is enough. Use very warm water, as hard as possible, on the sore arm if in acute pain, but whisper for your own variations often.

Try to not be scared while experimenting with the movements. Be positive even if you aggravate the pain, as you will know next time not to do it in that direction.

Tips

Keep *whispering*; for example, *"Soft. Don't contract. Just relax, sore arm. I love you. Let me lift you. Let me lift you completely."* Things like that! Sounds crazy, but who cares, as long as you prevent the freeze worsening?

The only way to stop the capsulitis at this stage is to keep the shoulder in its socket. As painful as lifting the arm can be, this exercise is one way to keep tissues stretching. The other very important movement is Shoulder CPR, which may be best performed under the shower simultaneously with this move.

The use of pain relief medication (as prescribed) may be necessary to perform some of the basic movements initially. Be tough enough to know when you need assistance from therapists, remedial gentle massage, Therapeutic Touch practitioners, or increased doses of pain medications.

As unbelievable as it sounds, as bad as your shoulder is today, it can get worse if attention is not given to the root cause of the pain. Ensure your attention remains on *whispering* for physical and emotional health. Remember the parable at the beginning of the book. These exercises work well if applied with the intent to heal.

"The shower was great, I knew that already, but the passive movements worked to get my hand up on the shower wall; then I could let the warm water run on the arm while doing the Shoulder CPR. I had to use the passive movement to get the arm back off the wall again. The passive lift like the picture was also my first way I could test the range of movement before and after new exercises. It needed more grip to lower it than raise it. Like you warned, on the way down it could easily catch if I was not concentrating . . . . Good improvements, though and faster than . . . . Thanks."—Adam

Shoulder CPR

This is one of the most successful exercises in the series. It is usually a very successful movement for alleviating pain and regaining shoulder alignment. It is very simple, but you have to work out the best angle for the arm each time. The following will guide you to be successful with this exercise. The simplicity and success of this exercise will make it your shoulder lifesaver!

Your arm is slightly different to anyone else's. This exercise will work well even with old and very painful shoulder restrictions. For some reason this movement also decreases stinging and pulsing pains. The compression pulsing movement realigns structures and decreases pain signals.

The familiar abbreviation CPR, for cardio-pulmonary resuscitation, is used here to emphasize the importance of resuscitating the shoulder position. **The movement done is similar to the pulsing motion used in actual CPR—short pulses and firm pressure, delivered with elbows locked straight.**

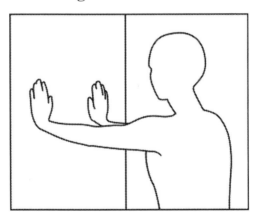

1. **Always assess your shoulder movements BEFORE exercise.** Often the quality of the movement improves first. This is felt by lifting the arm; assess how far it goes comfortably and also test how *light* it feels. Try to get used to assessing and noticing small variations; this

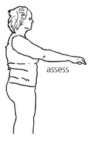

assess

will assist the *whispering* and help determine repetitions and hand position changes, etc. Use a roll of foam or towel to prevent wrist soreness if required.

2. Standing feet apart, facing a wall an arm's length away, raise your arm or arms (both to start with if possible).

3. Aim for about shoulder height.

4. If unable to reach that height yet, use your good arm to support your target arm and assist it to reach as high as possible on the wall; try angling your body for more effect (see YouTube demo).

5. If you are able to put two arms up, position them shoulder width apart (as illustrated). Keeping a slight lean into the wall, with body rigid and both arms locked straight, bounce into your wrist joints (if you can), like CPR, keeping the elbows locked straight, fingers pointing upward, and back straight. Repeat six to twelve short bounces initially and retest. Repeat often, performing up to forty Shoulder CPRs at a time. (Note: wrist needs to be okay, too.)

6. Remember, if you are doing two-handed Shoulder CPR, to maintain open arms with your wrists held in extension (as illustrated).

7. Get your wrists comfortable, as you must pulse or push through them. Use a hand towel or foam for extra support if needed.

8. Reassess your shoulder movements gently (once only for a guide on repetitions).

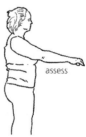

assess

Stop immediately if the movements have increased or aggravated any symptom. Alter to a side position before giving up as not workable for you (see variation below).

Post-Test: **Lift** your arm again over your head; assess if *you have* more movement, or perhaps it is less crunchy or feels smoother to move. Does it feel lighter? If you are not sure, pay more attention to the pretest angles, repeat the Shoulder CPR for the next few days, and see if pain or stinging in the shoulder area decreases. It should.

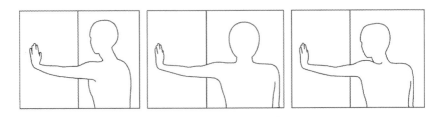

Variation

If doing the movement two handed had no immediate result, turn side-on and try six pulses, then reassess your ability to lift the arm. Many people with sore arms and very tight shoulder girdles find they have to begin *side-on, one arm* at a time first (see the middle illustration). This variation works well even in "hopeless" cases.

1.   Raise the affected arm as close to shoulder level as possible and try six pulses. Retest. It is very effective if combined with *whispering* to work out best angle for your shoulder.
2.   **Remember to assess before and after. Use this exercise doing four to eight times per day, with as many repetitions as *whispering* guides you to complete at each session** *eg just before you eat or drink.*
3.   One angle usually provides the best pain relief. You have to whisper to work that out for yourself.

Tips

Ideally, you should keep your arms level with your shoulder as you bounce the body into the wrists; the back should not arch or flex. If you cannot lift that high, try the side-on position first to ensure the joint directs itself back into its socket.

Do you have rounded shoulders? Again try side-on variations first; these work into the ball and socket better. You can also try the roller body exercise described at the end of this chapter if you are mobile enough.

Vary the way you lean in, as rhythm and depth of lean affects results.

This exercise is also a great pain reliever for throbbing shoulders or irritating pain in the front of the shoulder joint, as well as early rotator-cuff injuries and tenosynovitis (inflamed tendons).

This is an important exercise for minimizing contracting mechanisms within the capsular tissue. Repeat regularly.

When too painful on the wall alternative ideas exist

In shallow water. A similar movement can be achieved in a warm pool. One variation is to crawl on outstretched arms in shallow water. For example, use the children's pool (when it is not crowded), as it has a regular shallow depth. Allow your legs to just float passively behind you. An alternative is to stand in the shallow end of a regular pool, lean into the wall, and perform the CPR-style movements.

In a chair with armrests. Playing with the pulsing rhythm through the elbows, work out how to lean for best results. Try these steps using different positions (arm closer to your body, *whisper* best position):

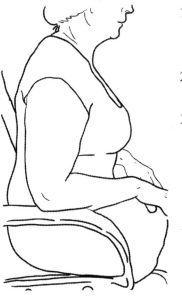

1. Assess your shoulder movement before and after six *pulses* (holding the same position).
2. Sit in a chair with armrests that suit you.
3. The hip joints must be behind your shoulder joints. (Look at the illustration and note the positioning of the hip joints behind the shoulder joints.)
5. Play with gently pushing down into the elbow in a pulsing manner. If the first position you choose causes soreness, vary it to suit your own arm.
5. Repeat a few times only, then reassess to gain certainty on the best direction of push and arm rest height and position.
6. Continue only if it feels nice or takes away pain.

The following story is an example of *whispering* and trying to get pain relief in a public place.

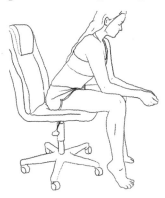

"I was seated and mindfully trying to shoulder whisper as the pain had started to build. I leant forward, putting my head into my hands, and whispered that my body will know how to stop the pulling pain soon . . . and I kept saying it, waiting, believing. Some moments went by before I realized what I was doing. The elbow had rested near my knee and my ankle was

moving up and down like a reverse Shoulder CPR (but through the elbow) movement. Just quietly. I then whispered my body would know the exact angle I need to move my shoulder too to optimize the pain relief. And it was really magical as I sensed to open my legs a little more, and instead of tapping the ankle, the heel raised and slower rhythm developed. The pain had already gone, but I had a feeling to continue for more repetitions. I understood this as more intense interventions for some other part of the body which I had not thought about. It is an awesome experience to have the body just do it. When I eventually sat back upright in the seat my whole neck and shoulder area was more even and relaxed."—Valerie

Passive Cradle across Chest

Pre-test assessment is not
essential for this movement, as
Passive Cradle Across Chest is for
pain relief rather than gaining
movement.

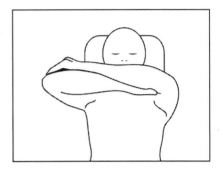

In a lying position, support
your affected arm fully by your
other arm in any way possible.
(See the illustration for one idea.)
Whisper for self-confidence; full passive support of the arm is less
painful. This movement introduces emotional healing and joint
stimulation. Sometimes it can feel very weird, so be patient.

While moving the forearm with the active arm try releasing any
hurt. Initially move it in a direction to please the shoulder, then pause
and use *whispering* to remind you to concentrate on letting love in.

Lower the arm any way you can without pain (try to hold it with the
stronger arm all the way back to its resting place). Repeat.

Advanced exercise

Support the arm thoroughly
as pictured and move the arm over
the chest in any direction *as long
as there is no forcing or pain*. The
more the arm moves toward the
head, the more the joint capsule
lengthens posteriorly. Determine
through *whispering* what is the best
movement for your current signs
and symptoms.

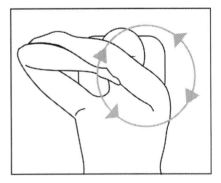

Tips

Do this gentle rhythmic movement perhaps twice a day.

Use gentle, rhythmic moves. Repeat as long as it is pleasurable and not "have-to-do-able." That is, don't do it if it is just one more chore or stressor in your life.

This is the safest way to get movement while lying, because you are holding and controlling, but remember to talk yourself into believing you are also identifying the emotional reasons for imbalance, too.

For this exercise, the more control you have over relaxing into the painful sensation and *whispering* to your body to guide you on which direction needs movement, the greater the success. If it hurts, move gently in another direction. Try giving the body every chance to settle into one movement.

Too painful?

If you are nervous and the pain is still acute, try it for one minute maximum. Throbbing within a few minutes is a reflection of new capsule position; be positive, and take pain relief medication if needed and as prescribed. Breathing postmovement is good instruction to yourself, allowing the tissue present to stretch and realign. "Enjoy the discomfort of healing" is another attitude to take. *Whisper*!

Hot showers postexercise can be effective and soothing. Remember again, your attitude toward the pain changes more neurotransmitters than any medical intervention. Keep positive about everything you are doing and feeling. It changes fast once initiated. Attempting different arm positions and rhythms may increase your ability to cope during the beginning period. Later on the most important thing is self-belief.

A correspondent sent this story to encourage some of my female participants to be a little stronger in their own self-belief.

"I was taught an exercise earlier on, swinging the arm downwards. It seems contrary to the idea of pushing the joint back into its socket as you describe. Nonetheless, as it was told to me by a medical practitioner I wasn't game to stop it. There was by and large no true effort on my part to engage in conversation with myself until after your treatment. Then the Shoulder CPRs and Passive Cradles made far more sense, and I experienced immediate changes in how I lifted my arm and night pain. Yet I continued with the doctor's exercise as well, but I had a nagging feeling it was a waste of time and undoing the other moves somewhat. As his appointment was approaching I felt a deep conditioning to do more of his exercises and override the intuitive feel of your (should I say my?) program. The night pain started to come back. I reported this at the appointment and got a steroid injection that day. I wonder now about the outcome if I had stood my ground and believed in my own ability more."—Pam

Froggy Exercise for Those Needing a Faster Result

The two exercises in the Froggy Series work simultaneously on the complex layers of tissues around the spine, fascia, neural tissue, and capsular layers of the shoulder. This is a great exercise for frozen shoulder and lower-back disorders. It additionally assists neural tissue length while activating new muscular sequences across the back and spine. The Froggy Series is wonderful for flexibility or pre-sport warm-up. It is particularly useful for teenagers prone to sitting for long periods during their growth spurts. There is a possibility of great success even with people with mild arthritic knees (gradually descending into the squat even though nervous and doubting their ability), and with youngsters with very tight hamstrings.

The Froggy Series is a strengthening-lengthening program. It is scary at first as it involves entering a deep squat position and being balanced (you may need to hold onto furniture that does not slide or tip while learning the exercise—see illustration). Balance and confidence comes with repetitions, so do not give up too early. *There are strict contraindications for this exercise. Read the warning box before starting (eg joint replacements etc.).*

Two phases

1. *Froggy-Balance:* Sliding off a lounge chair or couch into a deep squat, feet apart and turned outwards, and pushing into your arms to learn balance

2. *Froggy-Flop:* Pushing into your arms strongly and projecting your bottom backwards (not upwards) into a low chair or sofa behind you in a flopping action

Phase 1: Froggy-Balance

This is like the Shoulder CPR movement but in a deep squat.

Read the FULL safety box (page 81) before attempting this position and movement.

1. Assess your shoulder movements and pain scores.
2. Position into a *half-squat* position, on the floor, with a strong, stable chair behind you to prevent you from falling backwards. Some people prefer to start by sitting in a low chair or couch first and then sliding slowly off into a squat position, feet wide enough apart to have your shoulders and arms between your knees.

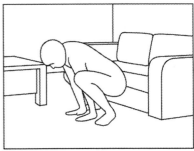

3. Place your hands on the floor (or on top of some books on the floor if you have larger or tight chest).
4. Rock forward onto your locked arms (again, the hands should be *between* the legs)
5. Rock back and forth into your straight, locked arms while learning your balance.
6. Return to the chair or couch. Sit still for a few minutes. Check how all the joints are feeling before standing and reassessing your movement.

Repeat two to four of these beginning froggy movements only. Sometimes the first time you will feel a little lightheaded from the new head-down position. Wait a few minutes before repeating, checking if everything is okay. Sometimes, even two rocks are enough for one day. You will work up to a greater level of tolerance.

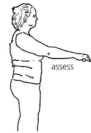

assess

Phase 2: Froggy-Flop

The second phase of pushing into the arms and then projecting *bottom first* back into the seat is tested and very popular; however, it requires more skill and initially many will doubt their ability to achieve it. The timing can be hard to grasp.

Do not Froggy-Flop if you—

- have hip or knee replacements
- have knee reconstructions or torn meniscus
- have instability of joint surfaces
- are six weeks or less postpartum
- your surgeon has not cleared you to do deep squats

Read the FULL safety box (page 81) before attempting this position and movement.

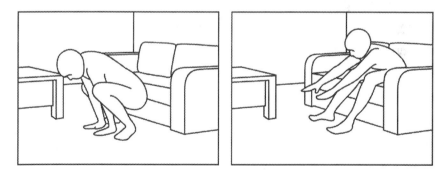

1. Check your arm movements first and ensure you are okay to squat!
2. Position yourself into the Froggy-Balance position, on the floor, with a strong, stable chair about a half a foot behind you. (The floor should not be slippery and the chair must be sturdy enough to prevent you from falling

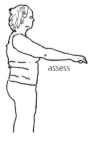

assess

backwards.) Place your feet in a comfortable position with your heels on the floor (as able).

3. Rock forward onto your straight arms (hands between legs) to warm up.

4. With your hands between your legs (or propped up on books or cushions), push down and try to project your bottom **backwards** into the chair without lifting it up into the air too high. Use the pressure through your arms to direct your bottom back into the chair.

5. You will literally land on your butt with a small plop.

6. Try to repeat it twice before reassessing your forward movement (called shoulder flexion). Vary your hand position to assess best results for your own aches and pains.

7. If improved, then whisper to decide if you need more, as it is new to many joints. Walk and assess, whisper how many per day is right for you. It is exciting how easy this can become over a few weeks. All housework and work activities become easier, so persist as you and only you can.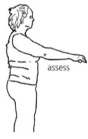

8. Reassess your shoulder flexion cautiously. (Be positive, okay?)

Safety for Doing Deep Squats

Do not do if it does not feel right.

Do not do postsurgery unless cleared to squat deeply by your surgeon.

Do not do if you are six weeks or less postpartum (childbirth).

Do not attempt if you have torn cartilage, worn menisci, or joint replacements (knees or hips)!

Older people take care—there are joints involved you have forgotten about!

Take care if you are overweight.

While care is required with sore or arthritic knees, stiff joints, and older back injuries there is a rhythm that develops in this exercise, using hamstrings at optimal range. With due caution you may be able to start at higher-level half-squat position and work down into a fuller squat over a few weeks. I have witnessed amazing results. Go slow, whisper often, and check the movement range changes frequently.

The chair must be solid, stable, and strong; ensure it cannot slide away.

Balance initially holding onto something solid. Take care, as many coffee tables will fall over.

Back pain sufferers can find this amazing or aggravating; try it initially slowly and in small numbers.

If you get dizzy, stop and follow the advice given below.

Dizzy?

If you become dizzy, check your blood pressure. New positions of the neck or head-down positions test the ability of your vestibular system, the system of balance monitored by your inner ear. If this is the primary cause of the dizziness, then it should decrease with gentle repetitions. Avoid doing this exercise in the heat. **Stop immediately if dizziness increases. Ask your medical practitioner for a full examination to discover the cause**. Can you reassure yourself it is okay? If not, see a doc. Or perhaps you have discovered something through *whispering* that may have gone unnoticed for a while. Have faith in your ongoing ability to improve.

Frequency

Try—
- absolutely none (0) for anyone who is too scared or absolutely in too much pain
- two froggy-flops for pre—and post-test assessment if trying this exercise the first time
- two froggy-flops for beginners
- two to three froggy-flops for experts

Be balanced and patient. You may need to do three Froggy-Balance tests before your first Froggy-Flop as a warm-up for the back and legs. **Some people feel a little sting in the deltoid area initially.** Others sense the grating of tendons in the capsule area. There should be no sharp or long-lasting pains anywhere. **The outcome testing is your best guide, rather than discomfort during the exercise.**

Pause after each Froggy-Flop, regain your balance fully, and then retest the arm movement. It should be no worse. Even if there is no initial gain in movement capacity it is very worthwhile repeating every other day for a while. Whisper for reassurance on this exercise, too.

"I freaked out with this one at first, as I got quite dizzy. Then I thought about it and said to myself that getting down on the floor is something I should be able to do. After repeating a few gentle Froggy-Balance movements (phase 1), the dizziness did not get worse. Two days later, I was game to try to advance with one Froggy-Flop and had no problems. I can

now do three of each without any symptoms only two weeks after starting. Oh, and the shoulder is heaps better too!"—Annie

"I read about this exercise and said no. My feet could not settle into position, I tipped backwards all the time and thought my knees would not get over the angle. Then I positioned two books under my hands, found a softer lower lounge that was really strong behind me. I still had to turn my feet out and do lots of warmups, but I eventually understood how the bum shoots into the chair by pushing through the arms first (i.e., not the head and shoulders hopping up). The results in the arm were amazing. Stung though at first. Thank you."—Carey

"I admit to being very skeptical of the froggy position, as I had not bent down like that for years. My children thought it was funny to watch, as I overbalanced often at the beginning and fell back into the lounge or on the rug. I persisted because my shoulder felt improved after doing the two trials. I can now do two Froggy-Balance warmups followed by three Froggy-Flops. The reason I am writing is to tell you that I have noticed that my house-duties like cleaning, mopping, and carrying groceries have also become pain-free since starting the Froggy-Flops. Thank you!"—Kay

Reassurance

This movement can feel awkward at first, and can make one feel impossibly fat and inflexible. Take the body to new heights and whisper to optimize improvements. If you are embarrassed by how silly you may look, try to impress others with your ingenious way of stretching so many organs and muscles with one move! Quietly get on with it, be better in your own self, and giggle more! Challenge your teenagers to repeat it as well as you! The movement can be viewed now on YouTube.

Troubleshooting

Sore wrists? Try any angle that is comfortable. Sometimes using a rolled-up hand towel or leaning onto books with your fingers over the edge can lessen wrist discomfort.

Sore back? Try one repetition, then walk around a little to assess if the movement has aggravated anything unduly. Surprisingly often, repeating a few times loosens the back.

Sore neck while in this position? Try changing the direction you are focusing on. Look more toward the floor or lengthen the back of the neck. Or vary upper-body position, and do not repeat more than once until tissue lengthens again. The tissue will stretch out in time.

Roller Body Work

These are an optional series of movements and related to the shoulder, thoracic spine, and hip joint juxtaposition. If you were to stand side-on and take a photograph of yourself in a natural position it should reveal a long slight curve in the thoracic area, and the hip and shoulder should be in a line. See the before-and-after pictures of the lady who spent four minutes on the roller as her first trial. Do you notice the difference in the shoulder angles? Even her cervical spine altered enough for her head to be in a better position etc.

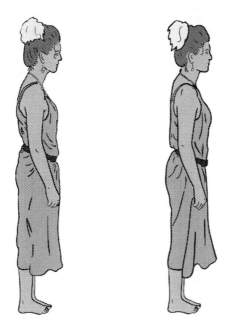

Trialing a roller can be fun, ensure not to jar arm when moving to and from the floor. Weight should be evenly distributed on the left and right sides and through the ankle joints.

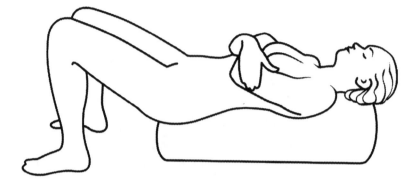

As strange as this exercise looks, it has incredible effects instantaneously on postural alignment. This assists numerous arm impairments as the shoulder joint can change position relative to the spine and thorax. I prefer you to take before and after photographs, side one, over a four week period. Do not study the image and become negative about yourself, this image is to encourage diligence in the rolling process and learn postural adjustments can be made naturally.

The roller has to be soft and firm at the same time. *It must be comfortable on your back for four minutes.* Hard PVC should be avoided; soft rollers are better, but not as fast in postural realignment. The general rule of thumb is if you have no padding on your spine then you need a softer roller. The length should at least as long as your trunk, covering head to bottom easily. The roller illustrated above is only just long enough. The bottom should not sink down or off the roller.

1. **Pre-test should be done now. Test your movements at shoulder, pain level, and quality of the movement in your whole body before lying down on the roller.**

2. Position your bottom on one end of the roller. Roll onto the roller with your head fully supported.

3. Lie however you are comfortable on your back on the roller for first trial. Most people simply hold their painful arm or prop it on pillows.

4. Retest your posture after 3 to 5 minutes on the roller either with photographs or by assessing your pain and freedom of movement.

5. Advance by trying different positions. Some common arm variations are offered here, but there are no rules for this when you are *whispering*—simply play around with it.

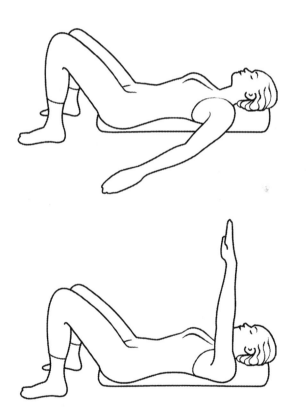

Tips

This movement can feel awkward at first, as it feels like you are doing nothing except lying there. Enjoy; it is the world's laziest and fastest exercise!

This is a great family exercise: check your teenager's posture, too. It is also good for anyone who has a tendency to believe they are rounded in the shoulders, or anyone who works primarily in a seated position.

Troubleshooting

Sore backbone? The roller is too hard or you are lying on it too long (four-minute maximum if you are slim-framed).

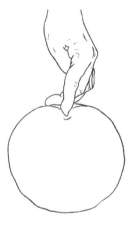

Sore arm after being on roller? The roller allowed the arm to position itself back into an awkward angle. Try readjusting with more support at arm next time (that is, if you are brave enough to try again) or simply repeat the most successful exercise so far to reduce symptoms (e.g., Shoulder CPR).

Having trouble finding a roller? You may be able to find a suitable roller at a physiotherapist or Pilates studio or from a foam manufacturer. Check online, too. The illustration shows how much the finger should compress into the dense foam to provide optimum comfort for your spine.

CHAPTER 8

THE 5 X 5 SERIES

That which is formed with personal experience is essentially alterable
and capable of being influenced by a new personal experience.
Moshe Feldenkrais (The Potent Self)

The 5 x 5 series is a *deterioration* prevention routine to be done
every day forever. This series is designed to prevent general wear
and tear, degeneration, and emotional sidetracks. The idea is to make
it practical to have these exercises become part of your lifestyle as soon
as you can.

The 5 x 5 series is quick to implement, easy to achieve, and applicable
in a variety of surroundings. Anyone who puts the family, work, and
friends before their own needs will find the 5 x 5 series worthwhile.
Consider how you brush and floss your teeth every day to prevent
decay. This is the same concept. As awful as decay sounds, it occurs in
other body parts, too, especially for middle-aged persons (usually 45+)
or anyone under a lot of stress.

The most important body parts and functions remain the upper body
and the ability to use your arms well, followed by the cardiac system.
Over and above this is your attitude or belief in your own SEL. The 5 x
5 series is for anyone too busy, too tired, or simply not interested in sport
or other highly physical activities.

The 5 x 5 series consists of —

1. Five pushups
2. Five sit-ups

3. Five minutes of jogging
4. Five minutes telling yourself how great you are
5. Five minutes asking for the greatest good for you

Do a trial for five days running, without judging yourself or feeling guilty over self-indulging, etc.

1. Pushups can be quarter or half pushups to start with. You can even start by standing and leaning into the kitchen counter. This is fun to do on soft surface, as it adds a little bounce and is softer on the knees. Stick to only five repetitions for at least a month. Don't advance until you get consistent with each part of the 5 x 5 series.

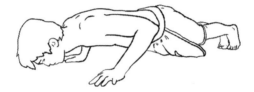

2. Sit-ups can be done in bed in the evening; mornings can be a little precarious with swollen joints and discs. Try with legs bent or straight to see what suits your own body best.

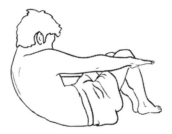

3. Running or jogging can be done outside the house first thing in the morning—then it is done! Often, the hardest thing to get your head around is that you only need five minutes (even

two minutes at the start). Safe, supporting shoes are a great idea, too.

4. Telling yourself how great you are is not to be based on what you have achieved. It has to be something you love about you. This can be hard to convince yourself on initially, but it is important to attract emotional SEL into the body that are loving you for who you are now. Try initially with the following statements as a guide:

- *I love my* _____ *(aspect of personality or character),*
- *I love my* _____ *(body part),*
- *I love my ability to* _____ *(personality/character again),*
- *I love the way my* _____ *(feature a body part again),* and
- *I love my* _____ *(a new one every time).*

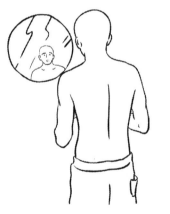

5. **Ask for the greatest good for you.** Can you ask that in a quiet place where any whispers bubbling from deep in the unconscious will be acknowledged? Meditation is like this if you are being guided for self-discovery. This is, after all, the essence of the *whispering*. It is different from affirmations and self-proclamations.

There is no need to go beyond this as the outside physical SEL uses these cues to self-heal without conscious understanding being necessary. However, do not feel limited to the statements above; make up more. Keep it up each day in any situation as you adapt to owning your SELf again.

The 5 x 5 series is a *decay*-prevention routine to be done every day forever. Follow it just like you follow your daily regime of brushing your teeth or doing pelvic floor exercises. If you are keen to do more as pain lessens, then my advice is to choose a sport or recreation you love. Refer to chapter 9 for a brief return-to-sport guide.

Guide yourself into believing more and more in the holistic elements of the 5 x 5 series from an injury-prevention viewpoint. It is almost too easy, yet boundless in its bounty.

CHAPTER 9

RETURN TO SPORT

There is no fear in love.
1 John: 4:18

Has your pain nearly gone? Is your arm movement restored? Is someone urging you to do more or return to an old sport? The important action is to begin with the 5 x 5 series first—stick with it for at least four weeks without any pain recurring, please. Return to sport only if you need to. Then if you are ready to start a new sport or exercise, you will find the following information very useful. Neuro Gym is a must for anyone completing sport training programs. It is similar to a foreshortened Feldenkrais™ awareness through movement exercise, only more prescriptive.

Start with Neuro Gym

The body has learned to help itself while you have been healing. For example, when you are standing, arms relaxed by your sides, the natural position is usually with the point of the elbow facing posteriorly (to the back) and your hands falling toward your thighs symmetrically.

Sometimes, muscles have assisted other shoulder muscles for too long and forget how to return to their old job. That makes *disbalance* ongoing and your shoulder potentially weaker than before. Some cute movements to quickly restore this follows.

Shoulder Blade Compensations

This can be worth taking a before-and-after photo of. The term *external rotation* means turning your arms out away from the body.

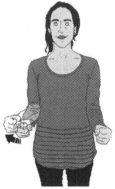

Phase 1

Arms by your side, bend the elbows to about eighty degrees and then talk to your body: *"I have to feel if I am moving muscles first between my shoulder blades while externally rotating my hand."*

Move the hands out and around sideways by using the muscles between the shoulder blades only, leaving your elbows in a relatively similar position. Repeat twice. Drop hands and relax.

Phase 2

Using the same starting position, pause and whisper; *"I have to move my shoulder the same way but without moving the shoulder blade muscles."* Repeat this movement two to five times gently, respecting your ability to ask for the movement.

The second movement should feel obviously different to the first. Retry the phase 1 exercise to check the difference.

It is not important which movement awareness dawns first. Sometimes, you may feel a warmth circulating down into the shoulder tendon that "woke up." No need to exercise this; it is an awakening whisper allowing the body to engage it again naturally. Repeat twice only.

Relax your arms and assess if you are aware of any variation in how the arms are hanging by your side now. For example, are the hands more symmetrical in their resting position, or is the direction the elbow points different from before? No need to repeat.

If you believe your postural habits reinstate the bad pattern, relief can be afforded with regular work on a soft roller.

The same checks should be done for each direction of movement in the arm.

What is occurring is that you are differentiating the shoulder ball and socket movement from the scapula or shoulder blade movements. In normal movement, both work in a rhythm and have a way of using the arm best suited to your own body's strength. That is why a fixed set of exercises for each movement should not be prescribed; it is specific to your personal needs and not the training method.

Try moving the arm in one direction (*eg forward and upwards, but not sideways*) by using three different muscle activations, see below for the most important variances:

1. The way you are doing it now.
2. Doing it attempting to hold the shoulder blade still or retracted/ backwards towards the spine.
3. Moving the arm forward only using the shoulder girdle and some neck muscles.

Whisper to your body through each variation of movement. It is not about correct or incorrect movement; it is simply altering neuronal pathways for a short burst.

You may notice, if you repeat step 1, that the body has adapted and accepted better movements naturally. So you must not be concerned with repeating any particular movement.

Depending on how old the injury is, the sequence may need to be repeated (e.g., every other day for a week) until you just *know* it is good enough for you.

Warmth is a signal that new tissues are adapting. Do not overwork this. It can be strong and surprising, as it often feels like you did hardly anything at all to provoke the sensation.

Strengthening More in Optimal Movement Patterns

Strengthening with weights too early can reinforce bad movement patterns. The encouraging thing with *whispering* is that once you and your body attune, you will be more likely to understand which muscle sequence needs strengthening, flexibility, or timing attention first.

However, the rehabilitation phase must include a strengthening component to maintain your health. The 5 x 5 series is optimal for this. It covers mental, physical, and emotional aspects of the condition, under your control through *whispering*. Most people choose walking first, but remember the 5 x 5 includes daily emotional and physical revision.

Tips

Care has to be exerted returning to sport, as it is amazing how quickly the strength and your original movement patterns change with pain. Perhaps a light Pilates routine for a month before returning to any sport would be a healthy (if affordable) choice.

Use awareness and control; tell the trainer if an area is hurting or excessively weak. No one should tell you to force through pain, as in this case it is a signal of tissue trauma.

Swimming

Avoid any stroke that stings, even dog-paddling. (Sting may suggest things are not right yet around the bursa.) Perhaps surprisingly, many find breaststroke the easiest stroke to return to first.

You should be able to introduce one exercise each session without fatigue. Ten minutes max! Wait and assess for night pain, and if none occurs, expand your routine. Take it slowly, but it is important to still do the 5 x 5 series first every day. Shoulder CPR is recommended for anyone with stings or random discomfort pre exercise and post.

Avoid freestyle for at least one month and until any sting at dog-paddling is completely gone. Ensure the 5 x 5 series is continued daily.

Gym Weights and Rigs

Keep away from any added weights on machines unless you were doing it every day before the injury and it is the same machine. Even then, just try a few that make you feel strong at first. The weakest area is often surprising, and those chest presses can do damage again, mainly to your fragile recovery rate. Your training in self-awareness, the 5 x 5 series, and *whispering* should by now recommend what machines to avoid, yet you will have to be stronger mentally to avoid private trainers telling you to push or do their reckoning on repetitions. This injury, even if fully recovered from emotional trauma, leaves a scar. Do not do anything anyone is telling you to do if it does not feel right, no matter what qualifications they hold.

Another tip: avoid gyms with lots of mirrors until you feel secure!

"At the hotel, I was all excited about having time away from family duties and doing some work on my shoulder at the hotel gym facilities. I had been working through the 5 x 5 at home and even though stronger wanted to try some old gym routines. The trouble was even though all my issues

with my emotional trauma were going OK, one look at myself in the gym's mirror made me hate everything about myself. My spirit was destroyed in an instant, and old negative self-talk bubbled to the surface. I was shocked to see me from different angles and how much weight I had piled on by eating my way out of the emotional trauma (pre-whispering!). So my only extra arm strengthening that trip was lifting a wine glass each night in my hotel room, sulking. After another day the 5 x 5 pulled me through with the positive self-talk returning and saying I am doing the best I am able given all that is. SO beware multi-angles mirrors too early, girls!"—So not giving my name!

Rubberized Stretching Bands and Devices

The concept behind exercises with rubber bands is to isolate and strengthen, for example the rotatory muscles. Do not do.

Even if you have a tear in your rotator cuff, all muscles work together, with synchronicity, for function.

If you have been told you have to train a muscle to take the tension off the one that is torn or inflamed, do so cautiously. Measure outcomes frequently and question any lack of result as politely as possible. If diagnosis is made based on an ultrasound examination, often very specific interventions of this character are advised. Be aware that ultrasounds are not always accurate diagnostically, while scans are. Specific or not, the tear occurred as a result of your natural functional movement patterns and postures. It is unlikely strength in one specific motor area changes neural linking. You need other moves for that.

RECOMMENDED READING

Molecules of Emotion: The Science behind Mind-Body Medicine, by Candace B. Pert (Simon & Schuster, 1999).

To Feel Good: The Science and Spirit of Bliss, by Candace B. Pert (Sounds True, 2007). Audio CD.

Waking the Tiger: Healing Trauma, by Peter A. Levine with Ann Frederick (North Atlantic Books, 1997).

The Biology of Belief: Unleashing the Power of Consciousness, Matter, & Miracles, by Bruce H. Lipton (Hay House, 2008).

Explain Pain, by David Butler and Lorimer Moseley (Orthopedic Physical Therapy Products, 2003).

Desiderata: A Poem for a Way of Life, by Max Ehrmann (Crown Publishers, 1995).

Therapeutic Touch Affects DNA Synthesis and Mineralization of Human Osteoblasts in Culture. Jhaveri, Ankur, Stephen Walsh, Yatzen Wang, MaryBeth McCarthy, Gloria Gronowicz. (Journal of Orthopaedic Research, 2008: 1541-1546).

APPENDIX A
ADDITIONAL BODY CHARTS

Pain Recording Chart

Date:

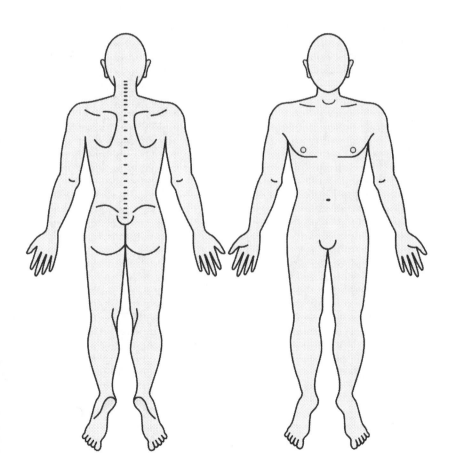

Pain Recording Chart

Date:

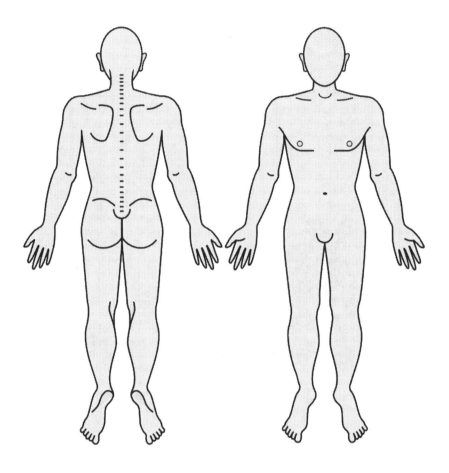

APPENDIX B

COMMENTS FROM CLIENTS

The faster you believe you are the strongest, most qualified person to change this shoulder problem, the faster the pain goes.

Care and attention to changing your mind matter most, as there are invariably a few habits that are not sound.

Here are some comments from clients:

"My left shoulder froze first, and I thought it was from lifting the wrong way, as all the therapists kept saying it was the biceps tendon. Yet after reading your book, I remembered around this time a severe emotional trauma that was so profound, it kept me in bed for a week. The shoulder pain turned into a freeze ten days after this . . . . I thought I must have slept on it the wrong way . . . . The emotional trauma subsided, but a similar emotional rejection came ten months after the first shoulder healed itself, and within one month, the good shoulder rapidly deteriorated, froze, etc."

"By the time I realized the pain was related to emotional issues, the freeze had begun despite rigorous therapy interventions . . . . Deep tissue massage therapy helped the secondary back pain, but nothing was helping the shoulder . . . ."

"In the end it was just better to work out the best exercises for my pain myself, based on the ones in the back of your book, of course. I took a little while trust myself about how many times to do each one, but now I understand why you don't say. Is it because it varies a bit each day? For example, yesterday was stressful, and usually having to do any extra

programs add more stress or guilt. So because I did not have to do fifteen sets of the exercises, etc., I was guilt free and still squeezed in the 5 x 5."

"I used the movements included in your book as a guide to gentler movements but still did one or two the therapists had prescribed already. But it was deciding about the emotional issues that were most important in recovery of my shoulder movement."

Are You Still Unsure?

A question often asked is this: "My doctor is recommending surgery for the pain, and I have not responded to physical therapy for six months. My arm aches every night, and I am not able to lift it anymore. Can I use this program, or should I have surgery?"

The answer is to comprehend your emotional trauma and ongoing stress and whether it relates to what the surgeon is going to operate on. The effect of hormonal factors remains unknown to date on surgery outcomes. However do not doubt a physical therapists ability to work on tissue. Yet it is not their job to diagnose hormonal *disbalances* or work on over-active emotional factors that are related to the condition.

A medical doctor or surgeon should not have any problems with you working through a DIY* self-healing intervention, to establish extent of hormonal, emotional or reactive related factors. It is after all for your greatest good.

---

* *DIY is an Australian expression for handypersons who 'Do It Yourself" around their own home*

APPENDIX C

TO THE PROFESSIONAL

The difficulty in producing a book of this type is to let go the requirement imposed on us professionally to say only what is evidence-based. In truth this book is a letting go of that requirement, but it is still founded on physiological principals and available research. It is different to other books on frozen shoulders as it encompasses thoughts relating to emotional events and physiologically associated responses.

The work in its original state came from my personal experiences with frozen shoulder first as a practitioner and then as a patient suffering more than the usual amount of pain and discomfort.

There is an expanding body of published research in this field, including links to hormonal *disbalances* and increased incidences of frozen shoulder (Hsu, et al., 2010) and there are moderate strength studies dealing with current practices relating to the treatment of frozen shoulder (Favejee, et al., 2011). Each individual study has its own slant, and outcomes tend to be based on the investigators' own beliefs. As natural as it is to spout such terms as *randomized* and *controlled*, we understand flaws in experimental design exist. There is often insufficient change in our technique over time to vary our belief in what works, but in the end frozen shoulder, and specifically primary frozen shoulder, has to date failed to have a fast or happy outcome for most of us.

Interestingly the content of this text was initially targeted for Google-savvy women who were over forty and unable to afford, access, or find treatments that assisted their pain or range of movement. As there remains limited clinical evidence on effective treatments and very limited evidence that any treatment is cost effective (Maund et al., 2012) an *open minded* state is to be recommended. The fact that this treatment approach also started to help others, including sports enthusiasts and elderly persons with other shoulder diagnoses, surprised.

Yet can recommending a simple self-help book be best practice for you? Is it viable in the long term to advise something that may decrease visitations to your clinic? While that ultimately is up to you, I would recommend excerpts that relate to gut feel and *whispering* as the experiment of choice, as ultimately surely one should *know* one's own body more than anyone else.

In the long term I hope this small book at least changes the way you initiate care. Altering your perception of a patient as a person who has acute shoulder pain to one who needs an integrative approach *with care* is a big step for practitioners. Even considering personal levels of output of energy toward a person who is in need of care, more compassion and understanding may just be efficient enough to bring about your own best practice time and time again. Nonetheless, it must be stated that ego can interfere, open eyes to your personal results of various populations groups, with and without potential cortisol changes, is a great start.

This book aims to define frozen shoulder as limbic, emotional, and chemical messenger related. The fact that I am suggesting this with very alternate and specific exercises contrary to the norm, should however, not affect anyone's ego, as once published it is after all available to adopt and quote. Basically do not criticize until you have lived through the process please and been to a good healer. Deliver it as yours as required, mine if you are skeptical, but then recommend my book. However in these cases, with this specific type of injury please do not ever condition yourself into believing that exercise matters over and above loving care. One without the other makes life unbearable.

BIBLIOGRAPHY

Many studies, systematic reviews and meta-analysis exist, here is one sample-

Buchbinder R, Green S, Youd JM, et al. 2006. Oral steroids for adhesive capsulitis. Cochrane Database Syst Rev; 4:CD006189.

Buchbinder R, Hoving JL, Green S, et al. 2004. Short course prednisolone for adhesive capsulitis (frozen shoulder or stiff painful shoulder): a randomised, double blind, placebo controlled trial. Ann Rheum Dis; 63:1460-9.

Favejee, M., Huisstede, H., and Koes, B., 2011. Frozen shoulder: the effectiveness of conservative and surgical interventions: systematic review, British Journal of Sports Medicine, Vol.45(1), p.49-5.

Hsu, J.E., Anakwenze, O., Warrenderb WJ., Abboud, JA., MD., 2010. Current review of adhesive capsulitis . J Shoulder Elbow Surg; 20, 502-514.

Hand C, Clipsham K, Rees JL, et al. 2008. Long-term outcome of frozen shoulder. J Shoulder Elbow Surg;17:231-6. 2.

Hand, G.C.R., Athanasou, N., Matthews, T and Carr A. J., 2007. The pathology of Frozen Shoulder. The Journal of Bone and Joitn Surgery, 89B (7), 928-932.

Hannafin JA, Chiaia TA. 2000. Adhesive capsulitis. A treatment approach. Clin Orthop Relat Res; 95-109. 3.

Kivimäki J, Pohjolainen T, Malmivaara A, et al. 2007. Manipulation under anesthesia with home exercises versus home exercises alone in the treatment of frozen shoulder: a randomized, controlled trial with 125 patients. J Shoulder Elbow Surg 2007;16:722-6.

Maund E, et al., 2012. Management of frozen shoulder: a systematic review and cost-effectiveness analysis. Health Technol Assess. 2012;16(11):1-264.

Pert, Candace.P., 1999 (Feb 17). Molecules of Emotion: The Science behind Mind-Body Medicine.

Ryans I, Montgomery A, Galway R, et al. 2005. A randomized controlled trial of intra—articular triamcinolone and/or physiotherapy in shoulder capsulitis. Rheumatology (Oxford); 44:529-35.

Tighe CB, Oakley WS Jr. 2008. The prevalence of a diabetic condition and adhesive capsulitis of the shoulder. South Med J.,101:591-5.